More Journals!

Want a Journal to give your busy friend or family member as a gift, or just want more Journal ideas?

Check out some of our other Journals...

Your Weekly Self Care Checklist
Gratitude Leaf: Creative Gratitude Journal
Weekly Better Health Checklist
Your Weekly Mental Health Checklist
Your Weekly Happiness Checklist
The Wheel of Life Workbook
The Positivity Workbook
Your Weekly Self Improvement Checklist

Choose from different lengths (60 days, 90 days and more) as well as different types of journals (with different goals and objectives). You are sure to find something that'll be great both as a personal journal and as a gift!

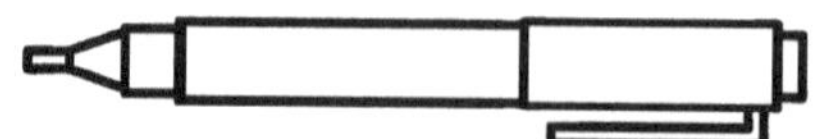

Free Gift!

Want a free gift?

Email us at
betterlifejournals@gmail.com

Title the email "Journal" and we will send you something fun!

Visit our website for more:
https://lifelabmagazine.com/better-life-journals/

YOUR WEEKLY BETTER SLEEP CHECKLIST

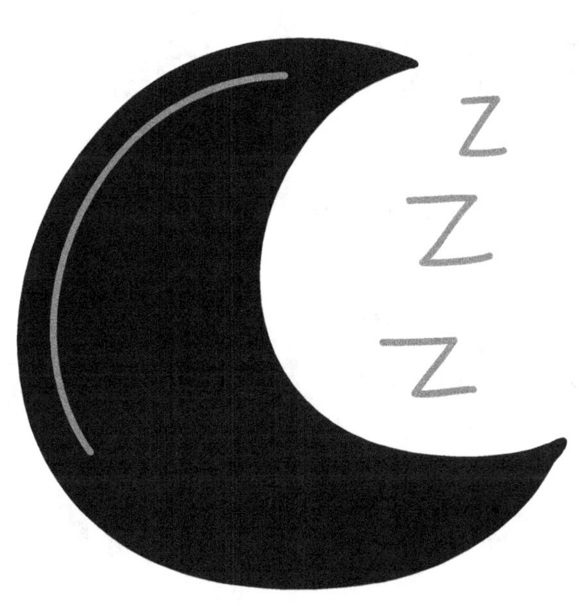

To keep the body in good health is a duty. otherwise we shall not be able to keep the mind strong and clear

BUDDHA

GETTING STARTED

The workbook and journal is pretty self-explanatory so you can just go through it at your own pace. That said, here are some tips that can help you get the most out of this:

- **Schedule a specific time** in the day when you will work on this workbook over the coming days. Having a specific time will help you stay on course. An easy way to do this is to schedule a recurring reminder on your phone's calendar.
- Start with the **Personal Assessment**.
- Next, work on the **healthy habit creator** section. This can help you create one good habit over the next 90 days, which will have a big impact on your wellbeing and happiness.
- Go through the **Wellbeing activities** list to get ideas for what you can do to take better care of yourself.
- Complete the journal pages every week (ideally daily) over the coming days. Take a bit of time before you get started to mentally prepare yourself if you need to but once you start, commit to doing them every day.

Most importantly, take it one day at a time. Small actions overtime will get you big results, as you will soon find out :)

Let's begin!

Good health is not something we can buy. However, it can be an extremely valuable savings account

ANNE WILSON SCHAEF

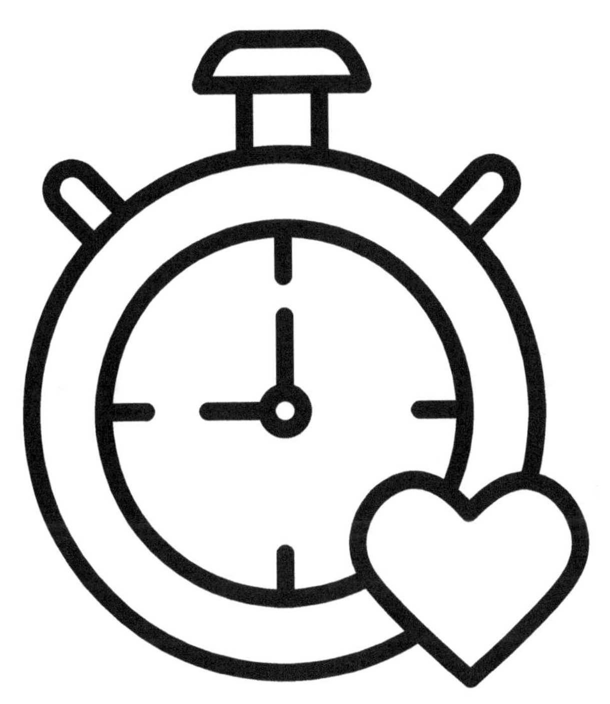

PERSONAL ASSESSMENT

1. What does getting good sleep mean to me?

2. What does me sleeping well regularly look like?

3. Current level of sleep   1 2 3 4 5

4. Desired level of sleep   1 2 3 4 5

PERSONAL ASSESSMENT

5. Why is it important for me to improve my sleep?

6. Who is the most healthy person I know, and what do I like most about them/their life?

7. What are the things I can do regularly to improve my sleep (both both big and small, like meditation and exercise)?

DECLARATION

I hereby commit to this daily practice.

Sign:

Date:

It is health that is the real wealth, and not pieces of gold and silver

MAHATMA GANDHI

HEALTHY HABIT CREATOR

Pick one small thing you can do every day for the next 90 days, something that will benefit your health (e.g. meditation, exercise, gratitude log, etc).

Once you have decided, use the habit tracker below to stick to this small daily positive habit by ticking/coloring one box for every day you practice the habit.

ONE THING = __________________________

1

30

60

90

To ensure good health: eat lightly, breathe deeply, live moderately, cultivate cheerfulness, and maintain an interest in life

WILLIAM LONDEN

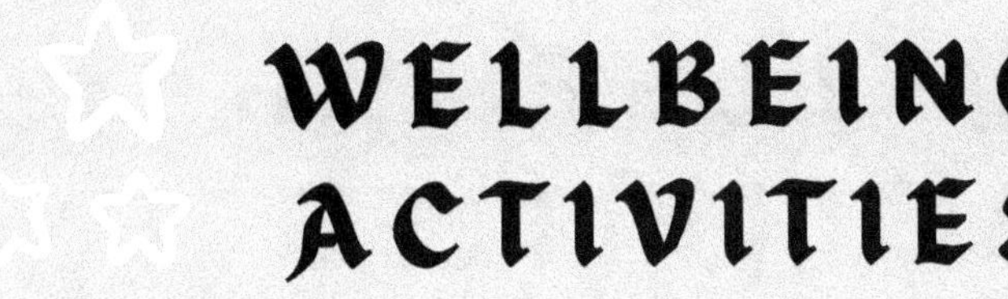

WELLBEING ACTIVITIES

Make a list of things that make you feel happy/good (we've included some ideas to get you started).

This list will come in very handy when planning your daily activities, and especially on days you aren't feeling so good (we all have off days, so it's ok).

○ Workout (even a 3-5 minutes of physical exercise can have a positive impact on your mood, and wellbeing)

○ Practice gratitude (practicing gratitude can not only help you feel good in the short term, but in the long term too!)

○ Meditation (practicing meditation can help you to regulate your emotions, and stress, better)

○ Random acts of kindness (being nice & helping others is one of the best ways, if not the best way, to feel joy)

○ Enjoy a nice cup of your favorite tea or coffee (even small things like this can have a big impact on your mood)

○

○

WELLBEING ACTIVITIES

In order to be the master of your life, you must first recognize that you are the rightful master of your brain, its owner and operator

ILCHI LEE

START YOUR JOURNEY!

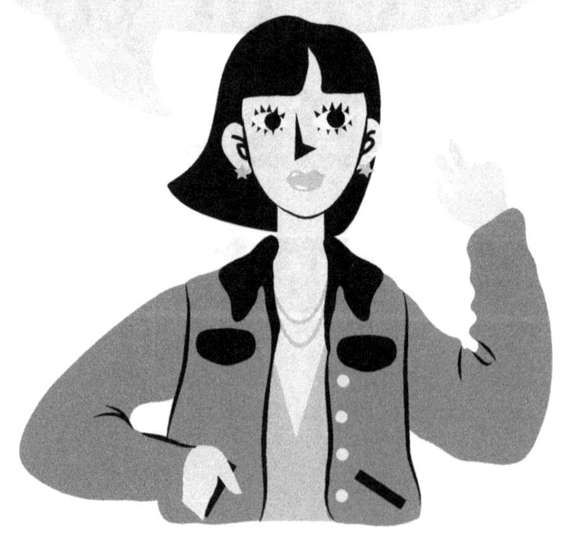

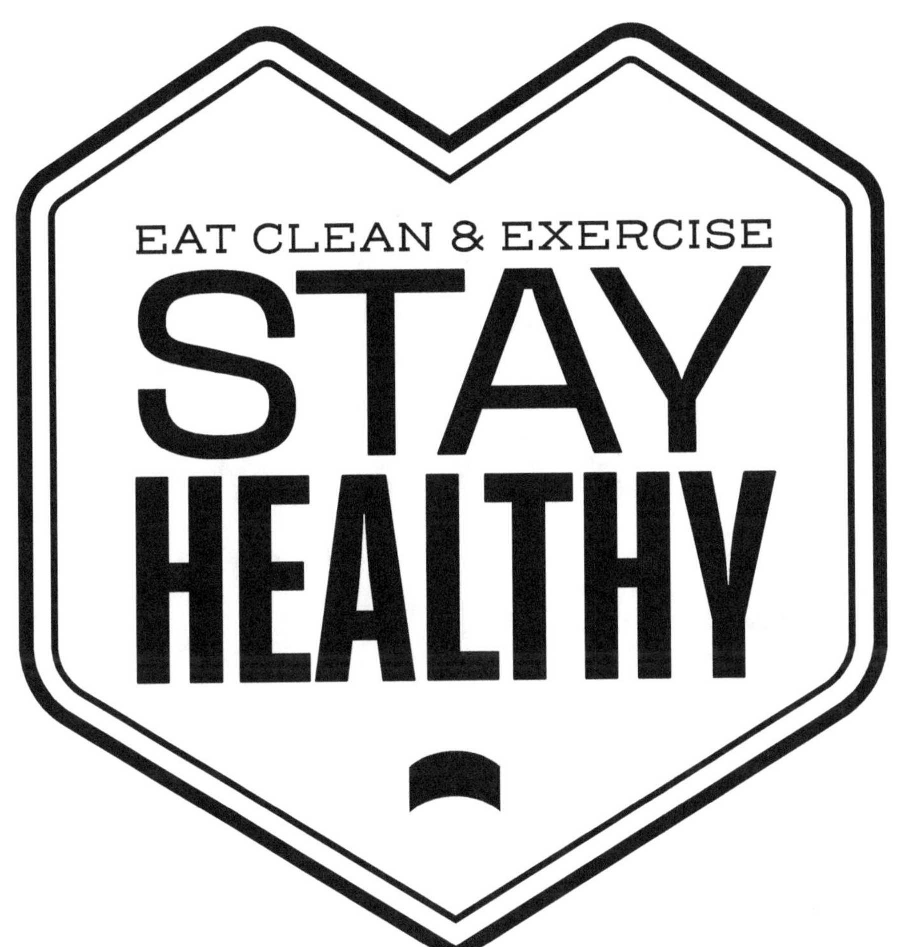

EAT CLEAN & EXERCISE
STAY
HEALTHY

MY PRIORITIES FOR THIS WEEK

GRATITUDE LOG

MAIN GOALS

DAILY ACTIVITIES

	M	T	W	T	F	S	S
Follow sleep routine	○	○	○	○	○	○	○
Avoid alcohol	○	○	○	○	○	○	○
Limit naps	○	○	○	○	○	○	○
Limit activities in bed	○	○	○	○	○	○	○
Exercise	○	○	○	○	○	○	○
Meditate	○	○	○	○	○	○	○
Journaling	○	○	○	○	○	○	○
No food late night	○	○	○	○	○	○	○
Shut off electronics in the evening	○	○	○	○	○	○	○
Less caffeine	○	○	○	○	○	○	○
Take magnesium	○	○	○	○	○	○	○

MY PRIORITIES FOR THIS WEEK

GRATITUDE LOG

MAIN GOALS

DAILY ACTIVITIES

	M	T	W	T	F	S	S
Follow sleep routine	○	○	○	○	○	○	○
Avoid alcohol	○	○	○	○	○	○	○
Limit naps	○	○	○	○	○	○	○
Limit activities in bed	○	○	○	○	○	○	○
Exercise	○	○	○	○	○	○	○
Meditate	○	○	○	○	○	○	○
Journaling	○	○	○	○	○	○	○
No food late night	○	○	○	○	○	○	○
Shut off electronics in the evening	○	○	○	○	○	○	○
Less caffeine	○	○	○	○	○	○	○
Take magnesium	○	○	○	○	○	○	○

MY PRIORITIES FOR THIS WEEK

GRATITUDE LOG

MAIN GOALS

DAILY ACTIVITIES

	M	T	W	T	F	S	S
Follow sleep routine	○	○	○	○	○	○	○
Avoid alcohol	○	○	○	○	○	○	○
Limit naps	○	○	○	○	○	○	○
Limit activities in bed	○	○	○	○	○	○	○
Exercise	○	○	○	○	○	○	○
Meditate	○	○	○	○	○	○	○
Journaling	○	○	○	○	○	○	○
No food late night	○	○	○	○	○	○	○
Shut off electronics in the evening	○	○	○	○	○	○	○
Less caffeine	○	○	○	○	○	○	○
Take magnesium	○	○	○	○	○	○	○

MY PRIORITIES FOR THIS WEEK

GRATITUDE LOG

MAIN GOALS

DAILY ACTIVITIES

	M	T	W	T	F	S	S
Follow sleep routine	○	○	○	○	○	○	○
Avoid alcohol	○	○	○	○	○	○	○
Limit naps	○	○	○	○	○	○	○
Limit activities in bed	○	○	○	○	○	○	○
Exercise	○	○	○	○	○	○	○
Meditate	○	○	○	○	○	○	○
Journaling	○	○	○	○	○	○	○
No food late night	○	○	○	○	○	○	○
Shut off electronics in the evening	○	○	○	○	○	○	○
Less caffeine	○	○	○	○	○	○	○
Take magnesium	○	○	○	○	○	○	○

MY PRIORITIES FOR THIS WEEK

GRATITUDE LOG

MAIN GOALS

DAILY ACTIVITIES

	M	T	W	T	F	S	S
Follow sleep routine	○	○	○	○	○	○	○
Avoid alcohol	○	○	○	○	○	○	○
Limit naps	○	○	○	○	○	○	○
Limit activities in bed	○	○	○	○	○	○	○
Exercise	○	○	○	○	○	○	○
Meditate	○	○	○	○	○	○	○
Journaling	○	○	○	○	○	○	○
No food late night	○	○	○	○	○	○	○
Shut off electronics in the evening	○	○	○	○	○	○	○
Less caffeine	○	○	○	○	○	○	○
Take magnesium	○	○	○	○	○	○	○

MY PRIORITIES FOR THIS WEEK

GRATITUDE LOG

MAIN GOALS

DAILY ACTIVITIES

	M	T	W	T	F	S	S
Follow sleep routine	○	○	○	○	○	○	○
Avoid alcohol	○	○	○	○	○	○	○
Limit naps	○	○	○	○	○	○	○
Limit activities in bed	○	○	○	○	○	○	○
Exercise	○	○	○	○	○	○	○
Meditate	○	○	○	○	○	○	○
Journaling	○	○	○	○	○	○	○
No food late night	○	○	○	○	○	○	○
Shut off electronics in the evening	○	○	○	○	○	○	○
Less caffeine	○	○	○	○	○	○	○
Take magnesium	○	○	○	○	○	○	○

MY PRIORITIES FOR THIS WEEK

GRATITUDE LOG

MAIN GOALS

DAILY ACTIVITIES

	M	T	W	T	F	S	S
Follow sleep routine	○	○	○	○	○	○	○
Avoid alcohol	○	○	○	○	○	○	○
Limit naps	○	○	○	○	○	○	○
Limit activities in bed	○	○	○	○	○	○	○
Exercise	○	○	○	○	○	○	○
Meditate	○	○	○	○	○	○	○
Journaling	○	○	○	○	○	○	○
No food late night	○	○	○	○	○	○	○
Shut off electronics in the evening	○	○	○	○	○	○	○
Less caffeine	○	○	○	○	○	○	○
Take magnesium	○	○	○	○	○	○	○

MY PRIORITIES FOR THIS WEEK

GRATITUDE LOG

MAIN GOALS

DAILY ACTIVITIES

	M	T	W	T	F	S	S
Follow sleep routine	○	○	○	○	○	○	○
Avoid alcohol	○	○	○	○	○	○	○
Limit naps	○	○	○	○	○	○	○
Limit activities in bed	○	○	○	○	○	○	○
Exercise	○	○	○	○	○	○	○
Meditate	○	○	○	○	○	○	○
Journaling	○	○	○	○	○	○	○
No food late night	○	○	○	○	○	○	○
Shut off electronics in the evening	○	○	○	○	○	○	○
Less caffeine	○	○	○	○	○	○	○
Take magnesium	○	○	○	○	○	○	○

MY PRIORITIES FOR THIS WEEK

GRATITUDE LOG

MAIN GOALS

DAILY ACTIVITIES

	M	T	W	T	F	S	S
Follow sleep routine	○	○	○	○	○	○	○
Avoid alcohol	○	○	○	○	○	○	○
Limit naps	○	○	○	○	○	○	○
Limit activities in bed	○	○	○	○	○	○	○
Exercise	○	○	○	○	○	○	○
Meditate	○	○	○	○	○	○	○
Journaling	○	○	○	○	○	○	○
No food late night	○	○	○	○	○	○	○
Shut off electronics in the evening	○	○	○	○	○	○	○
Less caffeine	○	○	○	○	○	○	○
Take magnesium	○	○	○	○	○	○	○

MY PRIORITIES FOR THIS WEEK

GRATITUDE LOG

MAIN GOALS

DAILY ACTIVITIES

	M	T	W	T	F	S	S
Follow sleep routine	○	○	○	○	○	○	○
Avoid alcohol	○	○	○	○	○	○	○
Limit naps	○	○	○	○	○	○	○
Limit activities in bed	○	○	○	○	○	○	○
Exercise	○	○	○	○	○	○	○
Meditate	○	○	○	○	○	○	○
Journaling	○	○	○	○	○	○	○
No food late night	○	○	○	○	○	○	○
Shut off electronics in the evening	○	○	○	○	○	○	○
Less caffeine	○	○	○	○	○	○	○
Take magnesium	○	○	○	○	○	○	○

MY PRIORITIES FOR THIS WEEK

GRATITUDE LOG

MAIN GOALS

DAILY ACTIVITIES

	M	T	W	T	F	S	S
Follow sleep routine	◯	◯	◯	◯	◯	◯	◯
Avoid alcohol	◯	◯	◯	◯	◯	◯	◯
Limit naps	◯	◯	◯	◯	◯	◯	◯
Limit activities in bed	◯	◯	◯	◯	◯	◯	◯
Exercise	◯	◯	◯	◯	◯	◯	◯
Meditate	◯	◯	◯	◯	◯	◯	◯
Journaling	◯	◯	◯	◯	◯	◯	◯
No food late night	◯	◯	◯	◯	◯	◯	◯
Shut off electronics in the evening	◯	◯	◯	◯	◯	◯	◯
Less caffeine	◯	◯	◯	◯	◯	◯	◯
Take magnesium	◯	◯	◯	◯	◯	◯	◯

MY PRIORITIES FOR THIS WEEK

GRATITUDE LOG

MAIN GOALS

DAILY ACTIVITIES

	M	T	W	T	F	S	S
Follow sleep routine	○	○	○	○	○	○	○
Avoid alcohol	○	○	○	○	○	○	○
Limit naps	○	○	○	○	○	○	○
Limit activities in bed	○	○	○	○	○	○	○
Exercise	○	○	○	○	○	○	○
Meditate	○	○	○	○	○	○	○
Journaling	○	○	○	○	○	○	○
No food late night	○	○	○	○	○	○	○
Shut off electronics in the evening	○	○	○	○	○	○	○
Less caffeine	○	○	○	○	○	○	○
Take magnesium	○	○	○	○	○	○	○

MY PRIORITIES FOR THIS WEEK

GRATITUDE LOG

MAIN GOALS

DAILY ACTIVITIES

	M	T	W	T	F	S	S
Follow sleep routine	○	○	○	○	○	○	○
Avoid alcohol	○	○	○	○	○	○	○
Limit naps	○	○	○	○	○	○	○
Limit activities in bed	○	○	○	○	○	○	○
Exercise	○	○	○	○	○	○	○
Meditate	○	○	○	○	○	○	○
Journaling	○	○	○	○	○	○	○
No food late night	○	○	○	○	○	○	○
Shut off electronics in the evening	○	○	○	○	○	○	○
Less caffeine	○	○	○	○	○	○	○
Take magnesium	○	○	○	○	○	○	○

MY PRIORITIES FOR THIS WEEK

GRATITUDE LOG

MAIN GOALS

DAILY ACTIVITIES

	M	T	W	T	F	S	S
Follow sleep routine	○	○	○	○	○	○	○
Avoid alcohol	○	○	○	○	○	○	○
Limit naps	○	○	○	○	○	○	○
Limit activities in bed	○	○	○	○	○	○	○
Exercise	○	○	○	○	○	○	○
Meditate	○	○	○	○	○	○	○
Journaling	○	○	○	○	○	○	○
No food late night	○	○	○	○	○	○	○
Shut off electronics in the evening	○	○	○	○	○	○	○
Less caffeine	○	○	○	○	○	○	○
Take magnesium	○	○	○	○	○	○	○

MY PRIORITIES FOR THIS WEEK

GRATITUDE LOG

MAIN GOALS

DAILY ACTIVITIES

	M	T	W	T	F	S	S
Follow sleep routine	○	○	○	○	○	○	○
Avoid alcohol	○	○	○	○	○	○	○
Limit naps	○	○	○	○	○	○	○
Limit activities in bed	○	○	○	○	○	○	○
Exercise	○	○	○	○	○	○	○
Meditate	○	○	○	○	○	○	○
Journaling	○	○	○	○	○	○	○
No food late night	○	○	○	○	○	○	○
Shut off electronics in the evening	○	○	○	○	○	○	○
Less caffeine	○	○	○	○	○	○	○
Take magnesium	○	○	○	○	○	○	○

MY PRIORITIES FOR THIS WEEK

GRATITUDE LOG

MAIN GOALS

DAILY ACTIVITIES

	M	T	W	T	F	S	S
Follow sleep routine	○	○	○	○	○	○	○
Avoid alcohol	○	○	○	○	○	○	○
Limit naps	○	○	○	○	○	○	○
Limit activities in bed	○	○	○	○	○	○	○
Exercise	○	○	○	○	○	○	○
Meditate	○	○	○	○	○	○	○
Journaling	○	○	○	○	○	○	○
No food late night	○	○	○	○	○	○	○
Shut off electronics in the evening	○	○	○	○	○	○	○
Less caffeine	○	○	○	○	○	○	○
Take magnesium	○	○	○	○	○	○	○

MY PRIORITIES FOR THIS WEEK

GRATITUDE LOG

MAIN GOALS

DAILY ACTIVITIES

	M	T	W	T	F	S	S
Follow sleep routine	○	○	○	○	○	○	○
Avoid alcohol	○	○	○	○	○	○	○
Limit naps	○	○	○	○	○	○	○
Limit activities in bed	○	○	○	○	○	○	○
Exercise	○	○	○	○	○	○	○
Meditate	○	○	○	○	○	○	○
Journaling	○	○	○	○	○	○	○
No food late night	○	○	○	○	○	○	○
Shut off electronics in the evening	○	○	○	○	○	○	○
Less caffeine	○	○	○	○	○	○	○
Take magnesium	○	○	○	○	○	○	○

MY PRIORITIES FOR THIS WEEK

GRATITUDE LOG

MAIN GOALS

DAILY ACTIVITIES

	M	T	W	T	F	S	S
Follow sleep routine	○	○	○	○	○	○	○
Avoid alcohol	○	○	○	○	○	○	○
Limit naps	○	○	○	○	○	○	○
Limit activities in bed	○	○	○	○	○	○	○
Exercise	○	○	○	○	○	○	○
Meditate	○	○	○	○	○	○	○
Journaling	○	○	○	○	○	○	○
No food late night	○	○	○	○	○	○	○
Shut off electronics in the evening	○	○	○	○	○	○	○
Less caffeine	○	○	○	○	○	○	○
Take magnesium	○	○	○	○	○	○	○

MY PRIORITIES FOR THIS WEEK

GRATITUDE LOG

MAIN GOALS

DAILY ACTIVITIES

	M	T	W	T	F	S	S
Follow sleep routine	○	○	○	○	○	○	○
Avoid alcohol	○	○	○	○	○	○	○
Limit naps	○	○	○	○	○	○	○
Limit activities in bed	○	○	○	○	○	○	○
Exercise	○	○	○	○	○	○	○
Meditate	○	○	○	○	○	○	○
Journaling	○	○	○	○	○	○	○
No food late night	○	○	○	○	○	○	○
Shut off electronics in the evening	○	○	○	○	○	○	○
Less caffeine	○	○	○	○	○	○	○
Take magnesium	○	○	○	○	○	○	○

MY PRIORITIES FOR THIS WEEK

GRATITUDE LOG

MAIN GOALS

DAILY ACTIVITIES

	M	T	W	T	F	S	S
Follow sleep routine	○	○	○	○	○	○	○
Avoid alcohol	○	○	○	○	○	○	○
Limit naps	○	○	○	○	○	○	○
Limit activities in bed	○	○	○	○	○	○	○
Exercise	○	○	○	○	○	○	○
Meditate	○	○	○	○	○	○	○
Journaling	○	○	○	○	○	○	○
No food late night	○	○	○	○	○	○	○
Shut off electronics in the evening	○	○	○	○	○	○	○
Less caffeine	○	○	○	○	○	○	○
Take magnesium	○	○	○	○	○	○	○

MY PRIORITIES FOR THIS WEEK

GRATITUDE LOG

MAIN GOALS

DAILY ACTIVITIES

	M	T	W	T	F	S	S
Follow sleep routine	○	○	○	○	○	○	○
Avoid alcohol	○	○	○	○	○	○	○
Limit naps	○	○	○	○	○	○	○
Limit activities in bed	○	○	○	○	○	○	○
Exercise	○	○	○	○	○	○	○
Meditate	○	○	○	○	○	○	○
Journaling	○	○	○	○	○	○	○
No food late night	○	○	○	○	○	○	○
Shut off electronics in the evening	○	○	○	○	○	○	○
Less caffeine	○	○	○	○	○	○	○
Take magnesium	○	○	○	○	○	○	○

MY PRIORITIES FOR THIS WEEK

GRATITUDE LOG

MAIN GOALS

DAILY ACTIVITIES

	M	T	W	T	F	S	S
Follow sleep routine	○	○	○	○	○	○	○
Avoid alcohol	○	○	○	○	○	○	○
Limit naps	○	○	○	○	○	○	○
Limit activities in bed	○	○	○	○	○	○	○
Exercise	○	○	○	○	○	○	○
Meditate	○	○	○	○	○	○	○
Journaling	○	○	○	○	○	○	○
No food late night	○	○	○	○	○	○	○
Shut off electronics in the evening	○	○	○	○	○	○	○
Less caffeine	○	○	○	○	○	○	○
Take magnesium	○	○	○	○	○	○	○

MY PRIORITIES FOR THIS WEEK

GRATITUDE LOG

MAIN GOALS

DAILY ACTIVITIES

	M	T	W	T	F	S	S
Follow sleep routine	○	○	○	○	○	○	○
Avoid alcohol	○	○	○	○	○	○	○
Limit naps	○	○	○	○	○	○	○
Limit activities in bed	○	○	○	○	○	○	○
Exercise	○	○	○	○	○	○	○
Meditate	○	○	○	○	○	○	○
Journaling	○	○	○	○	○	○	○
No food late night	○	○	○	○	○	○	○
Shut off electronics in the evening	○	○	○	○	○	○	○
Less caffeine	○	○	○	○	○	○	○
Take magnesium	○	○	○	○	○	○	○

MY PRIORITIES FOR THIS WEEK

GRATITUDE LOG

MAIN GOALS

DAILY ACTIVITIES

	M	T	W	T	F	S	S
Follow sleep routine	○	○	○	○	○	○	○
Avoid alcohol	○	○	○	○	○	○	○
Limit naps	○	○	○	○	○	○	○
Limit activities in bed	○	○	○	○	○	○	○
Exercise	○	○	○	○	○	○	○
Meditate	○	○	○	○	○	○	○
Journaling	○	○	○	○	○	○	○
No food late night	○	○	○	○	○	○	○
Shut off electronics in the evening	○	○	○	○	○	○	○
Less caffeine	○	○	○	○	○	○	○
Take magnesium	○	○	○	○	○	○	○

MY PRIORITIES FOR THIS WEEK

GRATITUDE LOG

MAIN GOALS

DAILY ACTIVITIES

	M	T	W	T	F	S	S
Follow sleep routine	○	○	○	○	○	○	○
Avoid alcohol	○	○	○	○	○	○	○
Limit naps	○	○	○	○	○	○	○
Limit activities in bed	○	○	○	○	○	○	○
Exercise	○	○	○	○	○	○	○
Meditate	○	○	○	○	○	○	○
Journaling	○	○	○	○	○	○	○
No food late night	○	○	○	○	○	○	○
Shut off electronics in the evening	○	○	○	○	○	○	○
Less caffeine	○	○	○	○	○	○	○
Take magnesium	○	○	○	○	○	○	○

MY PRIORITIES FOR THIS WEEK

GRATITUDE LOG

MAIN GOALS

DAILY ACTIVITIES

	M	T	W	T	F	S	S
Follow sleep routine	○	○	○	○	○	○	○
Avoid alcohol	○	○	○	○	○	○	○
Limit naps	○	○	○	○	○	○	○
Limit activities in bed	○	○	○	○	○	○	○
Exercise	○	○	○	○	○	○	○
Meditate	○	○	○	○	○	○	○
Journaling	○	○	○	○	○	○	○
No food late night	○	○	○	○	○	○	○
Shut off electronics in the evening	○	○	○	○	○	○	○
Less caffeine	○	○	○	○	○	○	○
Take magnesium	○	○	○	○	○	○	○

MY PRIORITIES FOR THIS WEEK

GRATITUDE LOG

MAIN GOALS

DAILY ACTIVITIES

	M	T	W	T	F	S	S
Follow sleep routine	○	○	○	○	○	○	○
Avoid alcohol	○	○	○	○	○	○	○
Limit naps	○	○	○	○	○	○	○
Limit activities in bed	○	○	○	○	○	○	○
Exercise	○	○	○	○	○	○	○
Meditate	○	○	○	○	○	○	○
Journaling	○	○	○	○	○	○	○
No food late night	○	○	○	○	○	○	○
Shut off electronics in the evening	○	○	○	○	○	○	○
Less caffeine	○	○	○	○	○	○	○
Take magnesium	○	○	○	○	○	○	○

MY PRIORITIES FOR THIS WEEK

GRATITUDE LOG

MAIN GOALS

DAILY ACTIVITIES

	M	T	W	T	F	S	S
Follow sleep routine	○	○	○	○	○	○	○
Avoid alcohol	○	○	○	○	○	○	○
Limit naps	○	○	○	○	○	○	○
Limit activities in bed	○	○	○	○	○	○	○
Exercise	○	○	○	○	○	○	○
Meditate	○	○	○	○	○	○	○
Journaling	○	○	○	○	○	○	○
No food late night	○	○	○	○	○	○	○
Shut off electronics in the evening	○	○	○	○	○	○	○
Less caffeine	○	○	○	○	○	○	○
Take magnesium	○	○	○	○	○	○	○

MY PRIORITIES FOR THIS WEEK

GRATITUDE LOG

MAIN GOALS

DAILY ACTIVITIES

	M	T	W	T	F	S	S
Follow sleep routine	○	○	○	○	○	○	○
Avoid alcohol	○	○	○	○	○	○	○
Limit naps	○	○	○	○	○	○	○
Limit activities in bed	○	○	○	○	○	○	○
Exercise	○	○	○	○	○	○	○
Meditate	○	○	○	○	○	○	○
Journaling	○	○	○	○	○	○	○
No food late night	○	○	○	○	○	○	○
Shut off electronics in the evening	○	○	○	○	○	○	○
Less caffeine	○	○	○	○	○	○	○
Take magnesium	○	○	○	○	○	○	○

MY PRIORITIES FOR THIS WEEK

GRATITUDE LOG

MAIN GOALS

DAILY ACTIVITIES

	M	T	W	T	F	S	S
Follow sleep routine	○	○	○	○	○	○	○
Avoid alcohol	○	○	○	○	○	○	○
Limit naps	○	○	○	○	○	○	○
Limit activities in bed	○	○	○	○	○	○	○
Exercise	○	○	○	○	○	○	○
Meditate	○	○	○	○	○	○	○
Journaling	○	○	○	○	○	○	○
No food late night	○	○	○	○	○	○	○
Shut off electronics in the evening	○	○	○	○	○	○	○
Less caffeine	○	○	○	○	○	○	○
Take magnesium	○	○	○	○	○	○	○

MY PRIORITIES FOR THIS WEEK

GRATITUDE LOG

MAIN GOALS

DAILY ACTIVITIES

	M	T	W	T	F	S	S
Follow sleep routine	○	○	○	○	○	○	○
Avoid alcohol	○	○	○	○	○	○	○
Limit naps	○	○	○	○	○	○	○
Limit activities in bed	○	○	○	○	○	○	○
Exercise	○	○	○	○	○	○	○
Meditate	○	○	○	○	○	○	○
Journaling	○	○	○	○	○	○	○
No food late night	○	○	○	○	○	○	○
Shut off electronics in the evening	○	○	○	○	○	○	○
Less caffeine	○	○	○	○	○	○	○
Take magnesium	○	○	○	○	○	○	○

MY PRIORITIES FOR THIS WEEK

GRATITUDE LOG

MAIN GOALS

DAILY ACTIVITIES

	M	T	W	T	F	S	S
Follow sleep routine	○	○	○	○	○	○	○
Avoid alcohol	○	○	○	○	○	○	○
Limit naps	○	○	○	○	○	○	○
Limit activities in bed	○	○	○	○	○	○	○
Exercise	○	○	○	○	○	○	○
Meditate	○	○	○	○	○	○	○
Journaling	○	○	○	○	○	○	○
No food late night	○	○	○	○	○	○	○
Shut off electronics in the evening	○	○	○	○	○	○	○
Less caffeine	○	○	○	○	○	○	○
Take magnesium	○	○	○	○	○	○	○

MY PRIORITIES FOR THIS WEEK

GRATITUDE LOG

MAIN GOALS

DAILY ACTIVITIES

	M	T	W	T	F	S	S
Follow sleep routine	○	○	○	○	○	○	○
Avoid alcohol	○	○	○	○	○	○	○
Limit naps	○	○	○	○	○	○	○
Limit activities in bed	○	○	○	○	○	○	○
Exercise	○	○	○	○	○	○	○
Meditate	○	○	○	○	○	○	○
Journaling	○	○	○	○	○	○	○
No food late night	○	○	○	○	○	○	○
Shut off electronics in the evening	○	○	○	○	○	○	○
Less caffeine	○	○	○	○	○	○	○
Take magnesium	○	○	○	○	○	○	○

MY PRIORITIES FOR THIS WEEK

GRATITUDE LOG

MAIN GOALS

DAILY ACTIVITIES

	M	T	W	T	F	S	S
Follow sleep routine	○	○	○	○	○	○	○
Avoid alcohol	○	○	○	○	○	○	○
Limit naps	○	○	○	○	○	○	○
Limit activities in bed	○	○	○	○	○	○	○
Exercise	○	○	○	○	○	○	○
Meditate	○	○	○	○	○	○	○
Journaling	○	○	○	○	○	○	○
No food late night	○	○	○	○	○	○	○
Shut off electronics in the evening	○	○	○	○	○	○	○
Less caffeine	○	○	○	○	○	○	○
Take magnesium	○	○	○	○	○	○	○

MY PRIORITIES FOR THIS WEEK

GRATITUDE LOG

MAIN GOALS

DAILY ACTIVITIES

	M	T	W	T	F	S	S
Follow sleep routine	○	○	○	○	○	○	○
Avoid alcohol	○	○	○	○	○	○	○
Limit naps	○	○	○	○	○	○	○
Limit activities in bed	○	○	○	○	○	○	○
Exercise	○	○	○	○	○	○	○
Meditate	○	○	○	○	○	○	○
Journaling	○	○	○	○	○	○	○
No food late night	○	○	○	○	○	○	○
Shut off electronics in the evening	○	○	○	○	○	○	○
Less caffeine	○	○	○	○	○	○	○
Take magnesium	○	○	○	○	○	○	○

MY PRIORITIES FOR THIS WEEK

GRATITUDE LOG

MAIN GOALS

DAILY ACTIVITIES

	M	T	W	T	F	S	S
Follow sleep routine	○	○	○	○	○	○	○
Avoid alcohol	○	○	○	○	○	○	○
Limit naps	○	○	○	○	○	○	○
Limit activities in bed	○	○	○	○	○	○	○
Exercise	○	○	○	○	○	○	○
Meditate	○	○	○	○	○	○	○
Journaling	○	○	○	○	○	○	○
No food late night	○	○	○	○	○	○	○
Shut off electronics in the evening	○	○	○	○	○	○	○
Less caffeine	○	○	○	○	○	○	○
Take magnesium	○	○	○	○	○	○	○

MY PRIORITIES FOR THIS WEEK

GRATITUDE LOG

MAIN GOALS

DAILY ACTIVITIES

	M	T	W	T	F	S	S
Follow sleep routine	○	○	○	○	○	○	○
Avoid alcohol	○	○	○	○	○	○	○
Limit naps	○	○	○	○	○	○	○
Limit activities in bed	○	○	○	○	○	○	○
Exercise	○	○	○	○	○	○	○
Meditate	○	○	○	○	○	○	○
Journaling	○	○	○	○	○	○	○
No food late night	○	○	○	○	○	○	○
Shut off electronics in the evening	○	○	○	○	○	○	○
Less caffeine	○	○	○	○	○	○	○
Take magnesium	○	○	○	○	○	○	○

MY PRIORITIES FOR THIS WEEK

GRATITUDE LOG

MAIN GOALS

DAILY ACTIVITIES

	M	T	W	T	F	S	S
Follow sleep routine	○	○	○	○	○	○	○
Avoid alcohol	○	○	○	○	○	○	○
Limit naps	○	○	○	○	○	○	○
Limit activities in bed	○	○	○	○	○	○	○
Exercise	○	○	○	○	○	○	○
Meditate	○	○	○	○	○	○	○
Journaling	○	○	○	○	○	○	○
No food late night	○	○	○	○	○	○	○
Shut off electronics in the evening	○	○	○	○	○	○	○
Less caffeine	○	○	○	○	○	○	○
Take magnesium	○	○	○	○	○	○	○

MY PRIORITIES FOR THIS WEEK

GRATITUDE LOG

MAIN GOALS

DAILY ACTIVITIES

	M	T	W	T	F	S	S
Follow sleep routine	○	○	○	○	○	○	○
Avoid alcohol	○	○	○	○	○	○	○
Limit naps	○	○	○	○	○	○	○
Limit activities in bed	○	○	○	○	○	○	○
Exercise	○	○	○	○	○	○	○
Meditate	○	○	○	○	○	○	○
Journaling	○	○	○	○	○	○	○
No food late night	○	○	○	○	○	○	○
Shut off electronics in the evening	○	○	○	○	○	○	○
Less caffeine	○	○	○	○	○	○	○
Take magnesium	○	○	○	○	○	○	○

MY PRIORITIES FOR THIS WEEK

GRATITUDE LOG

MAIN GOALS

DAILY ACTIVITIES

	M	T	W	T	F	S	S
Follow sleep routine	○	○	○	○	○	○	○
Avoid alcohol	○	○	○	○	○	○	○
Limit naps	○	○	○	○	○	○	○
Limit activities in bed	○	○	○	○	○	○	○
Exercise	○	○	○	○	○	○	○
Meditate	○	○	○	○	○	○	○
Journaling	○	○	○	○	○	○	○
No food late night	○	○	○	○	○	○	○
Shut off electronics in the evening	○	○	○	○	○	○	○
Less caffeine	○	○	○	○	○	○	○
Take magnesium	○	○	○	○	○	○	○

MY PRIORITIES FOR THIS WEEK

GRATITUDE LOG

MAIN GOALS

DAILY ACTIVITIES

	M	T	W	T	F	S	S
Follow sleep routine	○	○	○	○	○	○	○
Avoid alcohol	○	○	○	○	○	○	○
Limit naps	○	○	○	○	○	○	○
Limit activities in bed	○	○	○	○	○	○	○
Exercise	○	○	○	○	○	○	○
Meditate	○	○	○	○	○	○	○
Journaling	○	○	○	○	○	○	○
No food late night	○	○	○	○	○	○	○
Shut off electronics in the evening	○	○	○	○	○	○	○
Less caffeine	○	○	○	○	○	○	○
Take magnesium	○	○	○	○	○	○	○

MY PRIORITIES FOR THIS WEEK

GRATITUDE LOG

MAIN GOALS

DAILY ACTIVITIES

	M	T	W	T	F	S	S
Follow sleep routine	○	○	○	○	○	○	○
Avoid alcohol	○	○	○	○	○	○	○
Limit naps	○	○	○	○	○	○	○
Limit activities in bed	○	○	○	○	○	○	○
Exercise	○	○	○	○	○	○	○
Meditate	○	○	○	○	○	○	○
Journaling	○	○	○	○	○	○	○
No food late night	○	○	○	○	○	○	○
Shut off electronics in the evening	○	○	○	○	○	○	○
Less caffeine	○	○	○	○	○	○	○
Take magnesium	○	○	○	○	○	○	○

MY PRIORITIES FOR THIS WEEK

GRATITUDE LOG

MAIN GOALS

DAILY ACTIVITIES

	M	T	W	T	F	S	S
Follow sleep routine	○	○	○	○	○	○	○
Avoid alcohol	○	○	○	○	○	○	○
Limit naps	○	○	○	○	○	○	○
Limit activities in bed	○	○	○	○	○	○	○
Exercise	○	○	○	○	○	○	○
Meditate	○	○	○	○	○	○	○
Journaling	○	○	○	○	○	○	○
No food late night	○	○	○	○	○	○	○
Shut off electronics in the evening	○	○	○	○	○	○	○
Less caffeine	○	○	○	○	○	○	○
Take magnesium	○	○	○	○	○	○	○

MY PRIORITIES FOR THIS WEEK

GRATITUDE LOG

MAIN GOALS

DAILY ACTIVITIES

	M	T	W	T	F	S	S
Follow sleep routine	○	○	○	○	○	○	○
Avoid alcohol	○	○	○	○	○	○	○
Limit naps	○	○	○	○	○	○	○
Limit activities in bed	○	○	○	○	○	○	○
Exercise	○	○	○	○	○	○	○
Meditate	○	○	○	○	○	○	○
Journaling	○	○	○	○	○	○	○
No food late night	○	○	○	○	○	○	○
Shut off electronics in the evening	○	○	○	○	○	○	○
Less caffeine	○	○	○	○	○	○	○
Take magnesium	○	○	○	○	○	○	○

MY PRIORITIES FOR THIS WEEK

GRATITUDE LOG

MAIN GOALS

DAILY ACTIVITIES

	M	T	W	T	F	S	S
Follow sleep routine	○	○	○	○	○	○	○
Avoid alcohol	○	○	○	○	○	○	○
Limit naps	○	○	○	○	○	○	○
Limit activities in bed	○	○	○	○	○	○	○
Exercise	○	○	○	○	○	○	○
Meditate	○	○	○	○	○	○	○
Journaling	○	○	○	○	○	○	○
No food late night	○	○	○	○	○	○	○
Shut off electronics in the evening	○	○	○	○	○	○	○
Less caffeine	○	○	○	○	○	○	○
Take magnesium	○	○	○	○	○	○	○

MY PRIORITIES FOR THIS WEEK

GRATITUDE LOG

MAIN GOALS

DAILY ACTIVITIES

	M	T	W	T	F	S	S
Follow sleep routine	○	○	○	○	○	○	○
Avoid alcohol	○	○	○	○	○	○	○
Limit naps	○	○	○	○	○	○	○
Limit activities in bed	○	○	○	○	○	○	○
Exercise	○	○	○	○	○	○	○
Meditate	○	○	○	○	○	○	○
Journaling	○	○	○	○	○	○	○
No food late night	○	○	○	○	○	○	○
Shut off electronics in the evening	○	○	○	○	○	○	○
Less caffeine	○	○	○	○	○	○	○
Take magnesium	○	○	○	○	○	○	○

MY PRIORITIES FOR THIS WEEK

GRATITUDE LOG

MAIN GOALS

DAILY ACTIVITIES

	M	T	W	T	F	S	S
Follow sleep routine	◯	◯	◯	◯	◯	◯	◯
Avoid alcohol	◯	◯	◯	◯	◯	◯	◯
Limit naps	◯	◯	◯	◯	◯	◯	◯
Limit activities in bed	◯	◯	◯	◯	◯	◯	◯
Exercise	◯	◯	◯	◯	◯	◯	◯
Meditate	◯	◯	◯	◯	◯	◯	◯
Journaling	◯	◯	◯	◯	◯	◯	◯
No food late night	◯	◯	◯	◯	◯	◯	◯
Shut off electronics in the evening	◯	◯	◯	◯	◯	◯	◯
Less caffeine	◯	◯	◯	◯	◯	◯	◯
Take magnesium	◯	◯	◯	◯	◯	◯	◯

MY PRIORITIES FOR THIS WEEK

GRATITUDE LOG

MAIN GOALS

DAILY ACTIVITIES

	M	T	W	T	F	S	S
Follow sleep routine	○	○	○	○	○	○	○
Avoid alcohol	○	○	○	○	○	○	○
Limit naps	○	○	○	○	○	○	○
Limit activities in bed	○	○	○	○	○	○	○
Exercise	○	○	○	○	○	○	○
Meditate	○	○	○	○	○	○	○
Journaling	○	○	○	○	○	○	○
No food late night	○	○	○	○	○	○	○
Shut off electronics in the evening	○	○	○	○	○	○	○
Less caffeine	○	○	○	○	○	○	○
Take magnesium	○	○	○	○	○	○	○

MY PRIORITIES FOR THIS WEEK

GRATITUDE LOG

MAIN GOALS

DAILY ACTIVITIES

	M	T	W	T	F	S	S
Follow sleep routine	○	○	○	○	○	○	○
Avoid alcohol	○	○	○	○	○	○	○
Limit naps	○	○	○	○	○	○	○
Limit activities in bed	○	○	○	○	○	○	○
Exercise	○	○	○	○	○	○	○
Meditate	○	○	○	○	○	○	○
Journaling	○	○	○	○	○	○	○
No food late night	○	○	○	○	○	○	○
Shut off electronics in the evening	○	○	○	○	○	○	○
Less caffeine	○	○	○	○	○	○	○
Take magnesium	○	○	○	○	○	○	○

MY PRIORITIES FOR THIS WEEK

GRATITUDE LOG

MAIN GOALS

DAILY ACTIVITIES

	M	T	W	T	F	S	S
Follow sleep routine	○	○	○	○	○	○	○
Avoid alcohol	○	○	○	○	○	○	○
Limit naps	○	○	○	○	○	○	○
Limit activities in bed	○	○	○	○	○	○	○
Exercise	○	○	○	○	○	○	○
Meditate	○	○	○	○	○	○	○
Journaling	○	○	○	○	○	○	○
No food late night	○	○	○	○	○	○	○
Shut off electronics in the evening	○	○	○	○	○	○	○
Less caffeine	○	○	○	○	○	○	○
Take magnesium	○	○	○	○	○	○	○

MY PRIORITIES FOR THIS WEEK

GRATITUDE LOG

MAIN GOALS

DAILY ACTIVITIES

	M	T	W	T	F	S	S
Follow sleep routine	○	○	○	○	○	○	○
Avoid alcohol	○	○	○	○	○	○	○
Limit naps	○	○	○	○	○	○	○
Limit activities in bed	○	○	○	○	○	○	○
Exercise	○	○	○	○	○	○	○
Meditate	○	○	○	○	○	○	○
Journaling	○	○	○	○	○	○	○
No food late night	○	○	○	○	○	○	○
Shut off electronics in the evening	○	○	○	○	○	○	○
Less caffeine	○	○	○	○	○	○	○
Take magnesium	○	○	○	○	○	○	○

MY PRIORITIES FOR THIS WEEK

GRATITUDE LOG

MAIN GOALS

DAILY ACTIVITIES

	M	T	W	T	F	S	S
Follow sleep routine	○	○	○	○	○	○	○
Avoid alcohol	○	○	○	○	○	○	○
Limit naps	○	○	○	○	○	○	○
Limit activities in bed	○	○	○	○	○	○	○
Exercise	○	○	○	○	○	○	○
Meditate	○	○	○	○	○	○	○
Journaling	○	○	○	○	○	○	○
No food late night	○	○	○	○	○	○	○
Shut off electronics in the evening	○	○	○	○	○	○	○
Less caffeine	○	○	○	○	○	○	○
Take magnesium	○	○	○	○	○	○	○

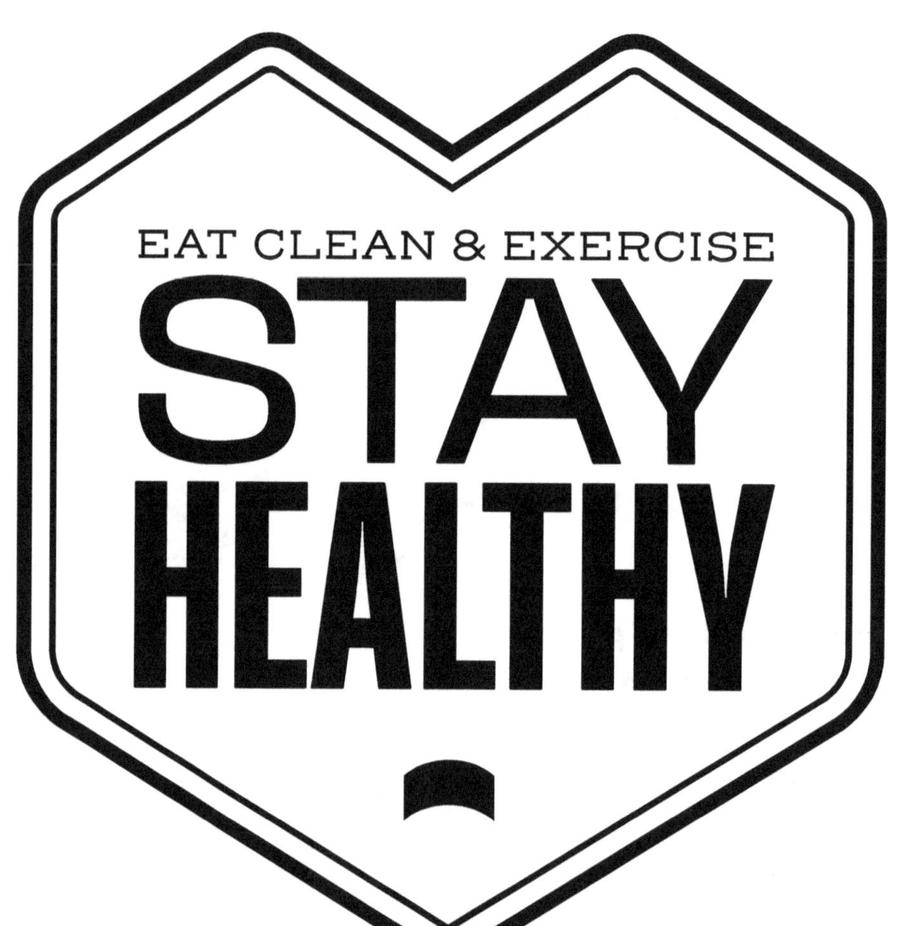
EAT CLEAN & EXERCISE
STAY
HEALTHY

MY PRIORITIES FOR THIS WEEK

GRATITUDE LOG

MAIN GOALS

DAILY ACTIVITIES

	M	T	W	T	F	S	S
Follow sleep routine	○	○	○	○	○	○	○
Avoid alcohol	○	○	○	○	○	○	○
Limit naps	○	○	○	○	○	○	○
Limit activities in bed	○	○	○	○	○	○	○
Exercise	○	○	○	○	○	○	○
Meditate	○	○	○	○	○	○	○
Journaling	○	○	○	○	○	○	○
No food late night	○	○	○	○	○	○	○
Shut off electronics in the evening	○	○	○	○	○	○	○
Less caffeine	○	○	○	○	○	○	○
Take magnesium	○	○	○	○	○	○	○

MY PRIORITIES FOR THIS WEEK

GRATITUDE LOG

MAIN GOALS

DAILY ACTIVITIES

	M	T	W	T	F	S	S
Follow sleep routine	○	○	○	○	○	○	○
Avoid alcohol	○	○	○	○	○	○	○
Limit naps	○	○	○	○	○	○	○
Limit activities in bed	○	○	○	○	○	○	○
Exercise	○	○	○	○	○	○	○
Meditate	○	○	○	○	○	○	○
Journaling	○	○	○	○	○	○	○
No food late night	○	○	○	○	○	○	○
Shut off electronics in the evening	○	○	○	○	○	○	○
Less caffeine	○	○	○	○	○	○	○
Take magnesium	○	○	○	○	○	○	○

MY PRIORITIES FOR THIS WEEK

GRATITUDE LOG

MAIN GOALS

DAILY ACTIVITIES

	M	T	W	T	F	S	S
Follow sleep routine	○	○	○	○	○	○	○
Avoid alcohol	○	○	○	○	○	○	○
Limit naps	○	○	○	○	○	○	○
Limit activities in bed	○	○	○	○	○	○	○
Exercise	○	○	○	○	○	○	○
Meditate	○	○	○	○	○	○	○
Journaling	○	○	○	○	○	○	○
No food late night	○	○	○	○	○	○	○
Shut off electronics in the evening	○	○	○	○	○	○	○
Less caffeine	○	○	○	○	○	○	○
Take magnesium	○	○	○	○	○	○	○

MY PRIORITIES FOR THIS WEEK

GRATITUDE LOG

MAIN GOALS

DAILY ACTIVITIES

	M	T	W	T	F	S	S
Follow sleep routine	○	○	○	○	○	○	○
Avoid alcohol	○	○	○	○	○	○	○
Limit naps	○	○	○	○	○	○	○
Limit activities in bed	○	○	○	○	○	○	○
Exercise	○	○	○	○	○	○	○
Meditate	○	○	○	○	○	○	○
Journaling	○	○	○	○	○	○	○
No food late night	○	○	○	○	○	○	○
Shut off electronics in the evening	○	○	○	○	○	○	○
Less caffeine	○	○	○	○	○	○	○
Take magnesium	○	○	○	○	○	○	○

MY PRIORITIES FOR THIS WEEK

GRATITUDE LOG

MAIN GOALS

DAILY ACTIVITIES

	M	T	W	T	F	S	S
Follow sleep routine	○	○	○	○	○	○	○
Avoid alcohol	○	○	○	○	○	○	○
Limit naps	○	○	○	○	○	○	○
Limit activities in bed	○	○	○	○	○	○	○
Exercise	○	○	○	○	○	○	○
Meditate	○	○	○	○	○	○	○
Journaling	○	○	○	○	○	○	○
No food late night	○	○	○	○	○	○	○
Shut off electronics in the evening	○	○	○	○	○	○	○
Less caffeine	○	○	○	○	○	○	○
Take magnesium	○	○	○	○	○	○	○

MY PRIORITIES FOR THIS WEEK

GRATITUDE LOG

MAIN GOALS

DAILY ACTIVITIES

	M	T	W	T	F	S	S
Follow sleep routine	○	○	○	○	○	○	○
Avoid alcohol	○	○	○	○	○	○	○
Limit naps	○	○	○	○	○	○	○
Limit activities in bed	○	○	○	○	○	○	○
Exercise	○	○	○	○	○	○	○
Meditate	○	○	○	○	○	○	○
Journaling	○	○	○	○	○	○	○
No food late night	○	○	○	○	○	○	○
Shut off electronics in the evening	○	○	○	○	○	○	○
Less caffeine	○	○	○	○	○	○	○
Take magnesium	○	○	○	○	○	○	○

MY PRIORITIES FOR THIS WEEK

GRATITUDE LOG

MAIN GOALS

DAILY ACTIVITIES

	M	T	W	T	F	S	S
Follow sleep routine	◯	◯	◯	◯	◯	◯	◯
Avoid alcohol	◯	◯	◯	◯	◯	◯	◯
Limit naps	◯	◯	◯	◯	◯	◯	◯
Limit activities in bed	◯	◯	◯	◯	◯	◯	◯
Exercise	◯	◯	◯	◯	◯	◯	◯
Meditate	◯	◯	◯	◯	◯	◯	◯
Journaling	◯	◯	◯	◯	◯	◯	◯
No food late night	◯	◯	◯	◯	◯	◯	◯
Shut off electronics in the evening	◯	◯	◯	◯	◯	◯	◯
Less caffeine	◯	◯	◯	◯	◯	◯	◯
Take magnesium	◯	◯	◯	◯	◯	◯	◯

MY PRIORITIES FOR THIS WEEK

GRATITUDE LOG

MAIN GOALS

DAILY ACTIVITIES

	M	T	W	T	F	S	S
Follow sleep routine	○	○	○	○	○	○	○
Avoid alcohol	○	○	○	○	○	○	○
Limit naps	○	○	○	○	○	○	○
Limit activities in bed	○	○	○	○	○	○	○
Exercise	○	○	○	○	○	○	○
Meditate	○	○	○	○	○	○	○
Journaling	○	○	○	○	○	○	○
No food late night	○	○	○	○	○	○	○
Shut off electronics in the evening	○	○	○	○	○	○	○
Less caffeine	○	○	○	○	○	○	○
Take magnesium	○	○	○	○	○	○	○

MY PRIORITIES FOR THIS WEEK

GRATITUDE LOG

MAIN GOALS

DAILY ACTIVITIES

	M	T	W	T	F	S	S
Follow sleep routine	○	○	○	○	○	○	○
Avoid alcohol	○	○	○	○	○	○	○
Limit naps	○	○	○	○	○	○	○
Limit activities in bed	○	○	○	○	○	○	○
Exercise	○	○	○	○	○	○	○
Meditate	○	○	○	○	○	○	○
Journaling	○	○	○	○	○	○	○
No food late night	○	○	○	○	○	○	○
Shut off electronics in the evening	○	○	○	○	○	○	○
Less caffeine	○	○	○	○	○	○	○
Take magnesium	○	○	○	○	○	○	○

MY PRIORITIES FOR THIS WEEK

GRATITUDE LOG

MAIN GOALS

DAILY ACTIVITIES

	M	T	W	T	F	S	S
Follow sleep routine	○	○	○	○	○	○	○
Avoid alcohol	○	○	○	○	○	○	○
Limit naps	○	○	○	○	○	○	○
Limit activities in bed	○	○	○	○	○	○	○
Exercise	○	○	○	○	○	○	○
Meditate	○	○	○	○	○	○	○
Journaling	○	○	○	○	○	○	○
No food late night	○	○	○	○	○	○	○
Shut off electronics in the evening	○	○	○	○	○	○	○
Less caffeine	○	○	○	○	○	○	○
Take magnesium	○	○	○	○	○	○	○

MY PRIORITIES FOR THIS WEEK

GRATITUDE LOG

MAIN GOALS

DAILY ACTIVITIES

	M	T	W	T	F	S	S
Follow sleep routine	◯	◯	◯	◯	◯	◯	◯
Avoid alcohol	◯	◯	◯	◯	◯	◯	◯
Limit naps	◯	◯	◯	◯	◯	◯	◯
Limit activities in bed	◯	◯	◯	◯	◯	◯	◯
Exercise	◯	◯	◯	◯	◯	◯	◯
Meditate	◯	◯	◯	◯	◯	◯	◯
Journaling	◯	◯	◯	◯	◯	◯	◯
No food late night	◯	◯	◯	◯	◯	◯	◯
Shut off electronics in the evening	◯	◯	◯	◯	◯	◯	◯
Less caffeine	◯	◯	◯	◯	◯	◯	◯
Take magnesium	◯	◯	◯	◯	◯	◯	◯

MY PRIORITIES FOR THIS WEEK

GRATITUDE LOG

MAIN GOALS

DAILY ACTIVITIES

	M	T	W	T	F	S	S
Follow sleep routine	○	○	○	○	○	○	○
Avoid alcohol	○	○	○	○	○	○	○
Limit naps	○	○	○	○	○	○	○
Limit activities in bed	○	○	○	○	○	○	○
Exercise	○	○	○	○	○	○	○
Meditate	○	○	○	○	○	○	○
Journaling	○	○	○	○	○	○	○
No food late night	○	○	○	○	○	○	○
Shut off electronics in the evening	○	○	○	○	○	○	○
Less caffeine	○	○	○	○	○	○	○
Take magnesium	○	○	○	○	○	○	○

MY PRIORITIES FOR THIS WEEK

GRATITUDE LOG

MAIN GOALS

DAILY ACTIVITIES

	M	T	W	T	F	S	S
Follow sleep routine	◯	◯	◯	◯	◯	◯	◯
Avoid alcohol	◯	◯	◯	◯	◯	◯	◯
Limit naps	◯	◯	◯	◯	◯	◯	◯
Limit activities in bed	◯	◯	◯	◯	◯	◯	◯
Exercise	◯	◯	◯	◯	◯	◯	◯
Meditate	◯	◯	◯	◯	◯	◯	◯
Journaling	◯	◯	◯	◯	◯	◯	◯
No food late night	◯	◯	◯	◯	◯	◯	◯
Shut off electronics in the evening	◯	◯	◯	◯	◯	◯	◯
Less caffeine	◯	◯	◯	◯	◯	◯	◯
Take magnesium	◯	◯	◯	◯	◯	◯	◯

MY PRIORITIES FOR THIS WEEK

GRATITUDE LOG

MAIN GOALS

DAILY ACTIVITIES

	M	T	W	T	F	S	S
Follow sleep routine	○	○	○	○	○	○	○
Avoid alcohol	○	○	○	○	○	○	○
Limit naps	○	○	○	○	○	○	○
Limit activities in bed	○	○	○	○	○	○	○
Exercise	○	○	○	○	○	○	○
Meditate	○	○	○	○	○	○	○
Journaling	○	○	○	○	○	○	○
No food late night	○	○	○	○	○	○	○
Shut off electronics in the evening	○	○	○	○	○	○	○
Less caffeine	○	○	○	○	○	○	○
Take magnesium	○	○	○	○	○	○	○

MY PRIORITIES FOR THIS WEEK

GRATITUDE LOG

MAIN GOALS

DAILY ACTIVITIES

	M	T	W	T	F	S	S
Follow sleep routine	◯	◯	◯	◯	◯	◯	◯
Avoid alcohol	◯	◯	◯	◯	◯	◯	◯
Limit naps	◯	◯	◯	◯	◯	◯	◯
Limit activities in bed	◯	◯	◯	◯	◯	◯	◯
Exercise	◯	◯	◯	◯	◯	◯	◯
Meditate	◯	◯	◯	◯	◯	◯	◯
Journaling	◯	◯	◯	◯	◯	◯	◯
No food late night	◯	◯	◯	◯	◯	◯	◯
Shut off electronics in the evening	◯	◯	◯	◯	◯	◯	◯
Less caffeine	◯	◯	◯	◯	◯	◯	◯
Take magnesium	◯	◯	◯	◯	◯	◯	◯

MY PRIORITIES FOR THIS WEEK

GRATITUDE LOG

MAIN GOALS

DAILY ACTIVITIES

	M	T	W	T	F	S	S
Follow sleep routine	○	○	○	○	○	○	○
Avoid alcohol	○	○	○	○	○	○	○
Limit naps	○	○	○	○	○	○	○
Limit activities in bed	○	○	○	○	○	○	○
Exercise	○	○	○	○	○	○	○
Meditate	○	○	○	○	○	○	○
Journaling	○	○	○	○	○	○	○
No food late night	○	○	○	○	○	○	○
Shut off electronics in the evening	○	○	○	○	○	○	○
Less caffeine	○	○	○	○	○	○	○
Take magnesium	○	○	○	○	○	○	○

MY PRIORITIES FOR THIS WEEK

GRATITUDE LOG

MAIN GOALS

DAILY ACTIVITIES

	M	T	W	T	F	S	S
Follow sleep routine	◯	◯	◯	◯	◯	◯	◯
Avoid alcohol	◯	◯	◯	◯	◯	◯	◯
Limit naps	◯	◯	◯	◯	◯	◯	◯
Limit activities in bed	◯	◯	◯	◯	◯	◯	◯
Exercise	◯	◯	◯	◯	◯	◯	◯
Meditate	◯	◯	◯	◯	◯	◯	◯
Journaling	◯	◯	◯	◯	◯	◯	◯
No food late night	◯	◯	◯	◯	◯	◯	◯
Shut off electronics in the evening	◯	◯	◯	◯	◯	◯	◯
Less caffeine	◯	◯	◯	◯	◯	◯	◯
Take magnesium	◯	◯	◯	◯	◯	◯	◯

MY PRIORITIES FOR THIS WEEK

GRATITUDE LOG

MAIN GOALS

DAILY ACTIVITIES

	M	T	W	T	F	S	S
Follow sleep routine	○	○	○	○	○	○	○
Avoid alcohol	○	○	○	○	○	○	○
Limit naps	○	○	○	○	○	○	○
Limit activities in bed	○	○	○	○	○	○	○
Exercise	○	○	○	○	○	○	○
Meditate	○	○	○	○	○	○	○
Journaling	○	○	○	○	○	○	○
No food late night	○	○	○	○	○	○	○
Shut off electronics in the evening	○	○	○	○	○	○	○
Less caffeine	○	○	○	○	○	○	○
Take magnesium	○	○	○	○	○	○	○

MY PRIORITIES FOR THIS WEEK

GRATITUDE LOG

MAIN GOALS

DAILY ACTIVITIES

	M	T	W	T	F	S	S
Follow sleep routine	○	○	○	○	○	○	○
Avoid alcohol	○	○	○	○	○	○	○
Limit naps	○	○	○	○	○	○	○
Limit activities in bed	○	○	○	○	○	○	○
Exercise	○	○	○	○	○	○	○
Meditate	○	○	○	○	○	○	○
Journaling	○	○	○	○	○	○	○
No food late night	○	○	○	○	○	○	○
Shut off electronics in the evening	○	○	○	○	○	○	○
Less caffeine	○	○	○	○	○	○	○
Take magnesium	○	○	○	○	○	○	○

MY PRIORITIES FOR THIS WEEK

GRATITUDE LOG

MAIN GOALS

DAILY ACTIVITIES

	M	T	W	T	F	S	S
Follow sleep routine	○	○	○	○	○	○	○
Avoid alcohol	○	○	○	○	○	○	○
Limit naps	○	○	○	○	○	○	○
Limit activities in bed	○	○	○	○	○	○	○
Exercise	○	○	○	○	○	○	○
Meditate	○	○	○	○	○	○	○
Journaling	○	○	○	○	○	○	○
No food late night	○	○	○	○	○	○	○
Shut off electronics in the evening	○	○	○	○	○	○	○
Less caffeine	○	○	○	○	○	○	○
Take magnesium	○	○	○	○	○	○	○

MY PRIORITIES FOR THIS WEEK

GRATITUDE LOG

MAIN GOALS

DAILY ACTIVITIES

	M	T	W	T	F	S	S
Follow sleep routine	○	○	○	○	○	○	○
Avoid alcohol	○	○	○	○	○	○	○
Limit naps	○	○	○	○	○	○	○
Limit activities in bed	○	○	○	○	○	○	○
Exercise	○	○	○	○	○	○	○
Meditate	○	○	○	○	○	○	○
Journaling	○	○	○	○	○	○	○
No food late night	○	○	○	○	○	○	○
Shut off electronics in the evening	○	○	○	○	○	○	○
Less caffeine	○	○	○	○	○	○	○
Take magnesium	○	○	○	○	○	○	○

MY PRIORITIES FOR THIS WEEK

GRATITUDE LOG

MAIN GOALS

DAILY ACTIVITIES

	M	T	W	T	F	S	S
Follow sleep routine	○	○	○	○	○	○	○
Avoid alcohol	○	○	○	○	○	○	○
Limit naps	○	○	○	○	○	○	○
Limit activities in bed	○	○	○	○	○	○	○
Exercise	○	○	○	○	○	○	○
Meditate	○	○	○	○	○	○	○
Journaling	○	○	○	○	○	○	○
No food late night	○	○	○	○	○	○	○
Shut off electronics in the evening	○	○	○	○	○	○	○
Less caffeine	○	○	○	○	○	○	○
Take magnesium	○	○	○	○	○	○	○

MY PRIORITIES FOR THIS WEEK

GRATITUDE LOG

MAIN GOALS

DAILY ACTIVITIES

	M	T	W	T	F	S	S
Follow sleep routine	○	○	○	○	○	○	○
Avoid alcohol	○	○	○	○	○	○	○
Limit naps	○	○	○	○	○	○	○
Limit activities in bed	○	○	○	○	○	○	○
Exercise	○	○	○	○	○	○	○
Meditate	○	○	○	○	○	○	○
Journaling	○	○	○	○	○	○	○
No food late night	○	○	○	○	○	○	○
Shut off electronics in the evening	○	○	○	○	○	○	○
Less caffeine	○	○	○	○	○	○	○
Take magnesium	○	○	○	○	○	○	○

WEEK OF:

MY PRIORITIES FOR THIS WEEK

GRATITUDE LOG

MAIN GOALS

DAILY ACTIVITIES

M T W T F S S

Follow sleep routine
Avoid alcohol
Limit naps
Limit activities in bed
Exercise
Meditate
Journaling
No food late night
Shut off electronics in the evening
Less caffeine
Take magnesium

MY PRIORITIES FOR THIS WEEK

GRATITUDE LOG

MAIN GOALS

DAILY ACTIVITIES

	M	T	W	T	F	S	S
Follow sleep routine	○	○	○	○	○	○	○
Avoid alcohol	○	○	○	○	○	○	○
Limit naps	○	○	○	○	○	○	○
Limit activities in bed	○	○	○	○	○	○	○
Exercise	○	○	○	○	○	○	○
Meditate	○	○	○	○	○	○	○
Journaling	○	○	○	○	○	○	○
No food late night	○	○	○	○	○	○	○
Shut off electronics in the evening	○	○	○	○	○	○	○
Less caffeine	○	○	○	○	○	○	○
Take magnesium	○	○	○	○	○	○	○

MY PRIORITIES FOR THIS WEEK

GRATITUDE LOG

MAIN GOALS

DAILY ACTIVITIES

	M	T	W	T	F	S	S
Follow sleep routine	○	○	○	○	○	○	○
Avoid alcohol	○	○	○	○	○	○	○
Limit naps	○	○	○	○	○	○	○
Limit activities in bed	○	○	○	○	○	○	○
Exercise	○	○	○	○	○	○	○
Meditate	○	○	○	○	○	○	○
Journaling	○	○	○	○	○	○	○
No food late night	○	○	○	○	○	○	○
Shut off electronics in the evening	○	○	○	○	○	○	○
Less caffeine	○	○	○	○	○	○	○
Take magnesium	○	○	○	○	○	○	○

MY PRIORITIES FOR THIS WEEK

GRATITUDE LOG

MAIN GOALS

DAILY ACTIVITIES

	M	T	W	T	F	S	S
Follow sleep routine	○	○	○	○	○	○	○
Avoid alcohol	○	○	○	○	○	○	○
Limit naps	○	○	○	○	○	○	○
Limit activities in bed	○	○	○	○	○	○	○
Exercise	○	○	○	○	○	○	○
Meditate	○	○	○	○	○	○	○
Journaling	○	○	○	○	○	○	○
No food late night	○	○	○	○	○	○	○
Shut off electronics in the evening	○	○	○	○	○	○	○
Less caffeine	○	○	○	○	○	○	○
Take magnesium	○	○	○	○	○	○	○

MY PRIORITIES FOR THIS WEEK

GRATITUDE LOG

MAIN GOALS

DAILY ACTIVITIES

	M	T	W	T	F	S	S
Follow sleep routine	○	○	○	○	○	○	○
Avoid alcohol	○	○	○	○	○	○	○
Limit naps	○	○	○	○	○	○	○
Limit activities in bed	○	○	○	○	○	○	○
Exercise	○	○	○	○	○	○	○
Meditate	○	○	○	○	○	○	○
Journaling	○	○	○	○	○	○	○
No food late night	○	○	○	○	○	○	○
Shut off electronics in the evening	○	○	○	○	○	○	○
Less caffeine	○	○	○	○	○	○	○
Take magnesium	○	○	○	○	○	○	○

MY PRIORITIES FOR THIS WEEK

GRATITUDE LOG

MAIN GOALS

DAILY ACTIVITIES

	M	T	W	T	F	S	S
Follow sleep routine	○	○	○	○	○	○	○
Avoid alcohol	○	○	○	○	○	○	○
Limit naps	○	○	○	○	○	○	○
Limit activities in bed	○	○	○	○	○	○	○
Exercise	○	○	○	○	○	○	○
Meditate	○	○	○	○	○	○	○
Journaling	○	○	○	○	○	○	○
No food late night	○	○	○	○	○	○	○
Shut off electronics in the evening	○	○	○	○	○	○	○
Less caffeine	○	○	○	○	○	○	○
Take magnesium	○	○	○	○	○	○	○

MY PRIORITIES FOR THIS WEEK

GRATITUDE LOG

MAIN GOALS

DAILY ACTIVITIES

	M	T	W	T	F	S	S
Follow sleep routine	○	○	○	○	○	○	○
Avoid alcohol	○	○	○	○	○	○	○
Limit naps	○	○	○	○	○	○	○
Limit activities in bed	○	○	○	○	○	○	○
Exercise	○	○	○	○	○	○	○
Meditate	○	○	○	○	○	○	○
Journaling	○	○	○	○	○	○	○
No food late night	○	○	○	○	○	○	○
Shut off electronics in the evening	○	○	○	○	○	○	○
Less caffeine	○	○	○	○	○	○	○
Take magnesium	○	○	○	○	○	○	○

MY PRIORITIES FOR THIS WEEK

GRATITUDE LOG

MAIN GOALS

DAILY ACTIVITIES

	M	T	W	T	F	S	S
Follow sleep routine	○	○	○	○	○	○	○
Avoid alcohol	○	○	○	○	○	○	○
Limit naps	○	○	○	○	○	○	○
Limit activities in bed	○	○	○	○	○	○	○
Exercise	○	○	○	○	○	○	○
Meditate	○	○	○	○	○	○	○
Journaling	○	○	○	○	○	○	○
No food late night	○	○	○	○	○	○	○
Shut off electronics in the evening	○	○	○	○	○	○	○
Less caffeine	○	○	○	○	○	○	○
Take magnesium	○	○	○	○	○	○	○

MY PRIORITIES FOR THIS WEEK

GRATITUDE LOG

MAIN GOALS

DAILY ACTIVITIES

	M	T	W	T	F	S	S
Follow sleep routine	○	○	○	○	○	○	○
Avoid alcohol	○	○	○	○	○	○	○
Limit naps	○	○	○	○	○	○	○
Limit activities in bed	○	○	○	○	○	○	○
Exercise	○	○	○	○	○	○	○
Meditate	○	○	○	○	○	○	○
Journaling	○	○	○	○	○	○	○
No food late night	○	○	○	○	○	○	○
Shut off electronics in the evening	○	○	○	○	○	○	○
Less caffeine	○	○	○	○	○	○	○
Take magnesium	○	○	○	○	○	○	○

MY PRIORITIES FOR THIS WEEK

GRATITUDE LOG

MAIN GOALS

DAILY ACTIVITIES

	M	T	W	T	F	S	S
Follow sleep routine	○	○	○	○	○	○	○
Avoid alcohol	○	○	○	○	○	○	○
Limit naps	○	○	○	○	○	○	○
Limit activities in bed	○	○	○	○	○	○	○
Exercise	○	○	○	○	○	○	○
Meditate	○	○	○	○	○	○	○
Journaling	○	○	○	○	○	○	○
No food late night	○	○	○	○	○	○	○
Shut off electronics in the evening	○	○	○	○	○	○	○
Less caffeine	○	○	○	○	○	○	○
Take magnesium	○	○	○	○	○	○	○

MY PRIORITIES FOR THIS WEEK

GRATITUDE LOG

MAIN GOALS

DAILY ACTIVITIES

	M	T	W	T	F	S	S
Follow sleep routine	◯	◯	◯	◯	◯	◯	◯
Avoid alcohol	◯	◯	◯	◯	◯	◯	◯
Limit naps	◯	◯	◯	◯	◯	◯	◯
Limit activities in bed	◯	◯	◯	◯	◯	◯	◯
Exercise	◯	◯	◯	◯	◯	◯	◯
Meditate	◯	◯	◯	◯	◯	◯	◯
Journaling	◯	◯	◯	◯	◯	◯	◯
No food late night	◯	◯	◯	◯	◯	◯	◯
Shut off electronics in the evening	◯	◯	◯	◯	◯	◯	◯
Less caffeine	◯	◯	◯	◯	◯	◯	◯
Take magnesium	◯	◯	◯	◯	◯	◯	◯

MY PRIORITIES FOR THIS WEEK

GRATITUDE LOG

MAIN GOALS

DAILY ACTIVITIES

	M	T	W	T	F	S	S
Follow sleep routine	○	○	○	○	○	○	○
Avoid alcohol	○	○	○	○	○	○	○
Limit naps	○	○	○	○	○	○	○
Limit activities in bed	○	○	○	○	○	○	○
Exercise	○	○	○	○	○	○	○
Meditate	○	○	○	○	○	○	○
Journaling	○	○	○	○	○	○	○
No food late night	○	○	○	○	○	○	○
Shut off electronics in the evening	○	○	○	○	○	○	○
Less caffeine	○	○	○	○	○	○	○
Take magnesium	○	○	○	○	○	○	○

MY PRIORITIES FOR THIS WEEK

GRATITUDE LOG

MAIN GOALS

DAILY ACTIVITIES

	M	T	W	T	F	S	S
Follow sleep routine	○	○	○	○	○	○	○
Avoid alcohol	○	○	○	○	○	○	○
Limit naps	○	○	○	○	○	○	○
Limit activities in bed	○	○	○	○	○	○	○
Exercise	○	○	○	○	○	○	○
Meditate	○	○	○	○	○	○	○
Journaling	○	○	○	○	○	○	○
No food late night	○	○	○	○	○	○	○
Shut off electronics in the evening	○	○	○	○	○	○	○
Less caffeine	○	○	○	○	○	○	○
Take magnesium	○	○	○	○	○	○	○

MY PRIORITIES FOR THIS WEEK

GRATITUDE LOG

MAIN GOALS

DAILY ACTIVITIES

	M	T	W	T	F	S	S
Follow sleep routine	○	○	○	○	○	○	○
Avoid alcohol	○	○	○	○	○	○	○
Limit naps	○	○	○	○	○	○	○
Limit activities in bed	○	○	○	○	○	○	○
Exercise	○	○	○	○	○	○	○
Meditate	○	○	○	○	○	○	○
Journaling	○	○	○	○	○	○	○
No food late night	○	○	○	○	○	○	○
Shut off electronics in the evening	○	○	○	○	○	○	○
Less caffeine	○	○	○	○	○	○	○
Take magnesium	○	○	○	○	○	○	○

MY PRIORITIES FOR THIS WEEK

GRATITUDE LOG

MAIN GOALS

DAILY ACTIVITIES

	M	T	W	T	F	S	S
Follow sleep routine	○	○	○	○	○	○	
Avoid alcohol	○	○	○	○	○	○	
Limit naps	○	○	○	○	○	○	
Limit activities in bed	○	○	○	○	○	○	
Exercise	○	○	○	○	○	○	
Meditate	○	○	○	○	○	○	
Journaling	○	○	○	○	○	○	
No food late night	○	○	○	○	○	○	
Shut off electronics in the evening	○	○	○	○	○	○	
Less caffeine	○	○	○	○	○	○	
Take magnesium	○	○	○	○	○	○	

MY PRIORITIES FOR THIS WEEK

GRATITUDE LOG

MAIN GOALS

DAILY ACTIVITIES

	M	T	W	T	F	S	S
Follow sleep routine	○	○	○	○	○	○	○
Avoid alcohol	○	○	○	○	○	○	○
Limit naps	○	○	○	○	○	○	○
Limit activities in bed	○	○	○	○	○	○	○
Exercise	○	○	○	○	○	○	○
Meditate	○	○	○	○	○	○	○
Journaling	○	○	○	○	○	○	○
No food late night	○	○	○	○	○	○	○
Shut off electronics in the evening	○	○	○	○	○	○	○
Less caffeine	○	○	○	○	○	○	○
Take magnesium	○	○	○	○	○	○	○

MY PRIORITIES FOR THIS WEEK

GRATITUDE LOG

MAIN GOALS

DAILY ACTIVITIES

	M	T	W	T	F	S	S
Follow sleep routine	○	○	○	○	○	○	○
Avoid alcohol	○	○	○	○	○	○	○
Limit naps	○	○	○	○	○	○	○
Limit activities in bed	○	○	○	○	○	○	○
Exercise	○	○	○	○	○	○	○
Meditate	○	○	○	○	○	○	○
Journaling	○	○	○	○	○	○	○
No food late night	○	○	○	○	○	○	○
Shut off electronics in the evening	○	○	○	○	○	○	○
Less caffeine	○	○	○	○	○	○	○
Take magnesium	○	○	○	○	○	○	○

MY PRIORITIES FOR THIS WEEK

GRATITUDE LOG

MAIN GOALS

DAILY ACTIVITIES

	M	T	W	T	F	S	S
Follow sleep routine	○	○	○	○	○	○	○
Avoid alcohol	○	○	○	○	○	○	○
Limit naps	○	○	○	○	○	○	○
Limit activities in bed	○	○	○	○	○	○	○
Exercise	○	○	○	○	○	○	○
Meditate	○	○	○	○	○	○	○
Journaling	○	○	○	○	○	○	○
No food late night	○	○	○	○	○	○	○
Shut off electronics in the evening	○	○	○	○	○	○	○
Less caffeine	○	○	○	○	○	○	○
Take magnesium	○	○	○	○	○	○	○

MY PRIORITIES FOR THIS WEEK

GRATITUDE LOG

MAIN GOALS

DAILY ACTIVITIES

	M	T	W	T	F	S	S
Follow sleep routine	○	○	○	○	○	○	○
Avoid alcohol	○	○	○	○	○	○	○
Limit naps	○	○	○	○	○	○	○
Limit activities in bed	○	○	○	○	○	○	○
Exercise	○	○	○	○	○	○	○
Meditate	○	○	○	○	○	○	○
Journaling	○	○	○	○	○	○	○
No food late night	○	○	○	○	○	○	○
Shut off electronics in the evening	○	○	○	○	○	○	○
Less caffeine	○	○	○	○	○	○	○
Take magnesium	○	○	○	○	○	○	○

MY PRIORITIES FOR THIS WEEK

GRATITUDE LOG

MAIN GOALS

DAILY ACTIVITIES

	M	T	W	T	F	S	S
Follow sleep routine	○	○	○	○	○	○	○
Avoid alcohol	○	○	○	○	○	○	○
Limit naps	○	○	○	○	○	○	○
Limit activities in bed	○	○	○	○	○	○	○
Exercise	○	○	○	○	○	○	○
Meditate	○	○	○	○	○	○	○
Journaling	○	○	○	○	○	○	○
No food late night	○	○	○	○	○	○	○
Shut off electronics in the evening	○	○	○	○	○	○	○
Less caffeine	○	○	○	○	○	○	○
Take magnesium	○	○	○	○	○	○	○

MY PRIORITIES FOR THIS WEEK

GRATITUDE LOG

MAIN GOALS

DAILY ACTIVITIES

	M	T	W	T	F	S	S
Follow sleep routine	○	○	○	○	○	○	○
Avoid alcohol	○	○	○	○	○	○	○
Limit naps	○	○	○	○	○	○	○
Limit activities in bed	○	○	○	○	○	○	○
Exercise	○	○	○	○	○	○	○
Meditate	○	○	○	○	○	○	○
Journaling	○	○	○	○	○	○	○
No food late night	○	○	○	○	○	○	○
Shut off electronics in the evening	○	○	○	○	○	○	○
Less caffeine	○	○	○	○	○	○	○
Take magnesium	○	○	○	○	○	○	○

MY PRIORITIES FOR THIS WEEK

GRATITUDE LOG

MAIN GOALS

DAILY ACTIVITIES

	M	T	W	T	F	S	S
Follow sleep routine	○	○	○	○	○	○	○
Avoid alcohol	○	○	○	○	○	○	○
Limit naps	○	○	○	○	○	○	○
Limit activities in bed	○	○	○	○	○	○	○
Exercise	○	○	○	○	○	○	○
Meditate	○	○	○	○	○	○	○
Journaling	○	○	○	○	○	○	○
No food late night	○	○	○	○	○	○	○
Shut off electronics in the evening	○	○	○	○	○	○	○
Less caffeine	○	○	○	○	○	○	○
Take magnesium	○	○	○	○	○	○	○

MY PRIORITIES FOR THIS WEEK

GRATITUDE LOG

MAIN GOALS

DAILY ACTIVITIES

	M	T	W	T	F	S	S
Follow sleep routine	○	○	○	○	○	○	○
Avoid alcohol	○	○	○	○	○	○	○
Limit naps	○	○	○	○	○	○	○
Limit activities in bed	○	○	○	○	○	○	○
Exercise	○	○	○	○	○	○	○
Meditate	○	○	○	○	○	○	○
Journaling	○	○	○	○	○	○	○
No food late night	○	○	○	○	○	○	○
Shut off electronics in the evening	○	○	○	○	○	○	○
Less caffeine	○	○	○	○	○	○	○
Take magnesium	○	○	○	○	○	○	○

MY PRIORITIES FOR THIS WEEK

GRATITUDE LOG

MAIN GOALS

DAILY ACTIVITIES

	M	T	W	T	F	S	S
Follow sleep routine	○	○	○	○	○	○	○
Avoid alcohol	○	○	○	○	○	○	○
Limit naps	○	○	○	○	○	○	○
Limit activities in bed	○	○	○	○	○	○	○
Exercise	○	○	○	○	○	○	○
Meditate	○	○	○	○	○	○	○
Journaling	○	○	○	○	○	○	○
No food late night	○	○	○	○	○	○	○
Shut off electronics in the evening	○	○	○	○	○	○	○
Less caffeine	○	○	○	○	○	○	○
Take magnesium	○	○	○	○	○	○	○

MY PRIORITIES FOR THIS WEEK

GRATITUDE LOG

MAIN GOALS

DAILY ACTIVITIES

	M	T	W	T	F	S	S
Follow sleep routine	○	○	○	○	○	○	○
Avoid alcohol	○	○	○	○	○	○	○
Limit naps	○	○	○	○	○	○	○
Limit activities in bed	○	○	○	○	○	○	○
Exercise	○	○	○	○	○	○	○
Meditate	○	○	○	○	○	○	○
Journaling	○	○	○	○	○	○	○
No food late night	○	○	○	○	○	○	○
Shut off electronics in the evening	○	○	○	○	○	○	○
Less caffeine	○	○	○	○	○	○	○
Take magnesium	○	○	○	○	○	○	○

MY PRIORITIES FOR THIS WEEK

GRATITUDE LOG

MAIN GOALS

DAILY ACTIVITIES

	M	T	W	T	F	S	S
Follow sleep routine	○	○	○	○	○	○	○
Avoid alcohol	○	○	○	○	○	○	○
Limit naps	○	○	○	○	○	○	○
Limit activities in bed	○	○	○	○	○	○	○
Exercise	○	○	○	○	○	○	○
Meditate	○	○	○	○	○	○	○
Journaling	○	○	○	○	○	○	○
No food late night	○	○	○	○	○	○	○
Shut off electronics in the evening	○	○	○	○	○	○	○
Less caffeine	○	○	○	○	○	○	○
Take magnesium	○	○	○	○	○	○	○

MY PRIORITIES FOR THIS WEEK

GRATITUDE LOG

MAIN GOALS

DAILY ACTIVITIES

	M	T	W	T	F	S	S
Follow sleep routine	○	○	○	○	○	○	○
Avoid alcohol	○	○	○	○	○	○	○
Limit naps	○	○	○	○	○	○	○
Limit activities in bed	○	○	○	○	○	○	○
Exercise	○	○	○	○	○	○	○
Meditate	○	○	○	○	○	○	○
Journaling	○	○	○	○	○	○	○
No food late night	○	○	○	○	○	○	○
Shut off electronics in the evening	○	○	○	○	○	○	○
Less caffeine	○	○	○	○	○	○	○
Take magnesium	○	○	○	○	○	○	○

MY PRIORITIES FOR THIS WEEK

GRATITUDE LOG

MAIN GOALS

DAILY ACTIVITIES

	M	T	W	T	F	S	S
Follow sleep routine	○	○	○	○	○	○	○
Avoid alcohol	○	○	○	○	○	○	○
Limit naps	○	○	○	○	○	○	○
Limit activities in bed	○	○	○	○	○	○	○
Exercise	○	○	○	○	○	○	○
Meditate	○	○	○	○	○	○	○
Journaling	○	○	○	○	○	○	○
No food late night	○	○	○	○	○	○	○
Shut off electronics in the evening	○	○	○	○	○	○	○
Less caffeine	○	○	○	○	○	○	○
Take magnesium	○	○	○	○	○	○	○

MY PRIORITIES FOR THIS WEEK

GRATITUDE LOG

MAIN GOALS

DAILY ACTIVITIES

	M	T	W	T	F	S	S
Follow sleep routine	○	○	○	○	○	○	○
Avoid alcohol	○	○	○	○	○	○	○
Limit naps	○	○	○	○	○	○	○
Limit activities in bed	○	○	○	○	○	○	○
Exercise	○	○	○	○	○	○	○
Meditate	○	○	○	○	○	○	○
Journaling	○	○	○	○	○	○	○
No food late night	○	○	○	○	○	○	○
Shut off electronics in the evening	○	○	○	○	○	○	○
Less caffeine	○	○	○	○	○	○	○
Take magnesium	○	○	○	○	○	○	○

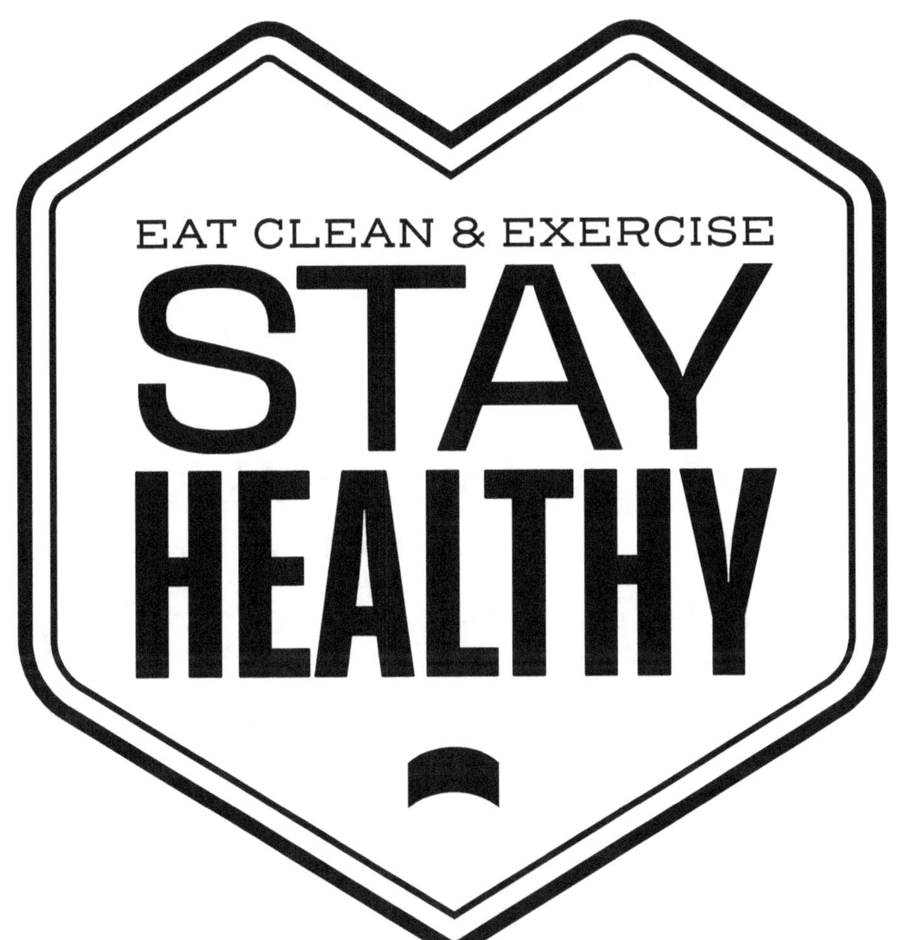

EAT CLEAN & EXERCISE
STAY
HEALTHY

MY PRIORITIES FOR THIS WEEK

GRATITUDE LOG

MAIN GOALS

DAILY ACTIVITIES

	M	T	W	T	F	S	S
Follow sleep routine	○	○	○	○	○	○	○
Avoid alcohol	○	○	○	○	○	○	○
Limit naps	○	○	○	○	○	○	○
Limit activities in bed	○	○	○	○	○	○	○
Exercise	○	○	○	○	○	○	○
Meditate	○	○	○	○	○	○	○
Journaling	○	○	○	○	○	○	○
No food late night	○	○	○	○	○	○	○
Shut off electronics in the evening	○	○	○	○	○	○	○
Less caffeine	○	○	○	○	○	○	○
Take magnesium	○	○	○	○	○	○	○

MY PRIORITIES FOR THIS WEEK

GRATITUDE LOG

MAIN GOALS

DAILY ACTIVITIES

	M	T	W	T	F	S	S
Follow sleep routine	○	○	○	○	○	○	○
Avoid alcohol	○	○	○	○	○	○	○
Limit naps	○	○	○	○	○	○	○
Limit activities in bed	○	○	○	○	○	○	○
Exercise	○	○	○	○	○	○	○
Meditate	○	○	○	○	○	○	○
Journaling	○	○	○	○	○	○	○
No food late night	○	○	○	○	○	○	○
Shut off electronics in the evening	○	○	○	○	○	○	○
Less caffeine	○	○	○	○	○	○	○
Take magnesium	○	○	○	○	○	○	○

MY PRIORITIES FOR THIS WEEK

GRATITUDE LOG

MAIN GOALS

DAILY ACTIVITIES

	M	T	W	T	F	S	S
Follow sleep routine	○	○	○	○	○	○	○
Avoid alcohol	○	○	○	○	○	○	○
Limit naps	○	○	○	○	○	○	○
Limit activities in bed	○	○	○	○	○	○	○
Exercise	○	○	○	○	○	○	○
Meditate	○	○	○	○	○	○	○
Journaling	○	○	○	○	○	○	○
No food late night	○	○	○	○	○	○	○
Shut off electronics in the evening	○	○	○	○	○	○	○
Less caffeine	○	○	○	○	○	○	○
Take magnesium	○	○	○	○	○	○	○

MY PRIORITIES FOR THIS WEEK

GRATITUDE LOG

MAIN GOALS

DAILY ACTIVITIES

	M	T	W	T	F	S	S
Follow sleep routine	◯	◯	◯	◯	◯	◯	◯
Avoid alcohol	◯	◯	◯	◯	◯	◯	◯
Limit naps	◯	◯	◯	◯	◯	◯	◯
Limit activities in bed	◯	◯	◯	◯	◯	◯	◯
Exercise	◯	◯	◯	◯	◯	◯	◯
Meditate	◯	◯	◯	◯	◯	◯	◯
Journaling	◯	◯	◯	◯	◯	◯	◯
No food late night	◯	◯	◯	◯	◯	◯	◯
Shut off electronics in the evening	◯	◯	◯	◯	◯	◯	◯
Less caffeine	◯	◯	◯	◯	◯	◯	◯
Take magnesium	◯	◯	◯	◯	◯	◯	◯

MY PRIORITIES FOR THIS WEEK

GRATITUDE LOG

MAIN GOALS

DAILY ACTIVITIES

	M	T	W	T	F	S	S
Follow sleep routine	○	○	○	○	○	○	○
Avoid alcohol	○	○	○	○	○	○	○
Limit naps	○	○	○	○	○	○	○
Limit activities in bed	○	○	○	○	○	○	○
Exercise	○	○	○	○	○	○	○
Meditate	○	○	○	○	○	○	○
Journaling	○	○	○	○	○	○	○
No food late night	○	○	○	○	○	○	○
Shut off electronics in the evening	○	○	○	○	○	○	○
Less caffeine	○	○	○	○	○	○	○
Take magnesium	○	○	○	○	○	○	○

MY PRIORITIES FOR THIS WEEK

GRATITUDE LOG

MAIN GOALS

DAILY ACTIVITIES

	M	T	W	T	F	S	S
Follow sleep routine	○	○	○	○	○	○	○
Avoid alcohol	○	○	○	○	○	○	○
Limit naps	○	○	○	○	○	○	○
Limit activities in bed	○	○	○	○	○	○	○
Exercise	○	○	○	○	○	○	○
Meditate	○	○	○	○	○	○	○
Journaling	○	○	○	○	○	○	○
No food late night	○	○	○	○	○	○	○
Shut off electronics in the evening	○	○	○	○	○	○	○
Less caffeine	○	○	○	○	○	○	○
Take magnesium	○	○	○	○	○	○	○

MY PRIORITIES FOR THIS WEEK

GRATITUDE LOG

MAIN GOALS

DAILY ACTIVITIES

	M	T	W	T	F	S	S
Follow sleep routine	○	○	○	○	○	○	○
Avoid alcohol	○	○	○	○	○	○	○
Limit naps	○	○	○	○	○	○	○
Limit activities in bed	○	○	○	○	○	○	○
Exercise	○	○	○	○	○	○	○
Meditate	○	○	○	○	○	○	○
Journaling	○	○	○	○	○	○	○
No food late night	○	○	○	○	○	○	○
Shut off electronics in the evening	○	○	○	○	○	○	○
Less caffeine	○	○	○	○	○	○	○
Take magnesium	○	○	○	○	○	○	○

MY PRIORITIES FOR THIS WEEK

GRATITUDE LOG

MAIN GOALS

DAILY ACTIVITIES

	M	T	W	T	F	S	S
Follow sleep routine	◯	◯	◯	◯	◯	◯	◯
Avoid alcohol	◯	◯	◯	◯	◯	◯	◯
Limit naps	◯	◯	◯	◯	◯	◯	◯
Limit activities in bed	◯	◯	◯	◯	◯	◯	◯
Exercise	◯	◯	◯	◯	◯	◯	◯
Meditate	◯	◯	◯	◯	◯	◯	◯
Journaling	◯	◯	◯	◯	◯	◯	◯
No food late night	◯	◯	◯	◯	◯	◯	◯
Shut off electronics in the evening	◯	◯	◯	◯	◯	◯	◯
Less caffeine	◯	◯	◯	◯	◯	◯	◯
Take magnesium	◯	◯	◯	◯	◯	◯	◯

MY PRIORITIES FOR THIS WEEK

GRATITUDE LOG

MAIN GOALS

DAILY ACTIVITIES

	M	T	W	T	F	S	S
Follow sleep routine	○	○	○	○	○	○	○
Avoid alcohol	○	○	○	○	○	○	○
Limit naps	○	○	○	○	○	○	○
Limit activities in bed	○	○	○	○	○	○	○
Exercise	○	○	○	○	○	○	○
Meditate	○	○	○	○	○	○	○
Journaling	○	○	○	○	○	○	○
No food late night	○	○	○	○	○	○	○
Shut off electronics in the evening	○	○	○	○	○	○	○
Less caffeine	○	○	○	○	○	○	○
Take magnesium	○	○	○	○	○	○	○

MY PRIORITIES FOR THIS WEEK

GRATITUDE LOG

MAIN GOALS

DAILY ACTIVITIES

	M	T	W	T	F	S	S
Follow sleep routine	○	○	○	○	○	○	○
Avoid alcohol	○	○	○	○	○	○	○
Limit naps	○	○	○	○	○	○	○
Limit activities in bed	○	○	○	○	○	○	○
Exercise	○	○	○	○	○	○	○
Meditate	○	○	○	○	○	○	○
Journaling	○	○	○	○	○	○	○
No food late night	○	○	○	○	○	○	○
Shut off electronics in the evening	○	○	○	○	○	○	○
Less caffeine	○	○	○	○	○	○	○
Take magnesium	○	○	○	○	○	○	○

MY PRIORITIES FOR THIS WEEK

GRATITUDE LOG

MAIN GOALS

DAILY ACTIVITIES

	M	T	W	T	F	S	S
Follow sleep routine	○	○	○	○	○	○	○
Avoid alcohol	○	○	○	○	○	○	○
Limit naps	○	○	○	○	○	○	○
Limit activities in bed	○	○	○	○	○	○	○
Exercise	○	○	○	○	○	○	○
Meditate	○	○	○	○	○	○	○
Journaling	○	○	○	○	○	○	○
No food late night	○	○	○	○	○	○	○
Shut off electronics in the evening	○	○	○	○	○	○	○
Less caffeine	○	○	○	○	○	○	○
Take magnesium	○	○	○	○	○	○	○

MY PRIORITIES FOR THIS WEEK

GRATITUDE LOG

MAIN GOALS

DAILY ACTIVITIES

	M	T	W	T	F	S	S
Follow sleep routine	○	○	○	○	○	○	○
Avoid alcohol	○	○	○	○	○	○	○
Limit naps	○	○	○	○	○	○	○
Limit activities in bed	○	○	○	○	○	○	○
Exercise	○	○	○	○	○	○	○
Meditate	○	○	○	○	○	○	○
Journaling	○	○	○	○	○	○	○
No food late night	○	○	○	○	○	○	○
Shut off electronics in the evening	○	○	○	○	○	○	○
Less caffeine	○	○	○	○	○	○	○
Take magnesium	○	○	○	○	○	○	○

MY PRIORITIES FOR THIS WEEK

GRATITUDE LOG

MAIN GOALS

DAILY ACTIVITIES

	M	T	W	T	F	S	S
Follow sleep routine	○	○	○	○	○	○	○
Avoid alcohol	○	○	○	○	○	○	○
Limit naps	○	○	○	○	○	○	○
Limit activities in bed	○	○	○	○	○	○	○
Exercise	○	○	○	○	○	○	○
Meditate	○	○	○	○	○	○	○
Journaling	○	○	○	○	○	○	○
No food late night	○	○	○	○	○	○	○
Shut off electronics in the evening	○	○	○	○	○	○	○
Less caffeine	○	○	○	○	○	○	○
Take magnesium	○	○	○	○	○	○	○

MY PRIORITIES FOR THIS WEEK

GRATITUDE LOG

MAIN GOALS

DAILY ACTIVITIES

	M	T	W	T	F	S	S
Follow sleep routine	○	○	○	○	○	○	○
Avoid alcohol	○	○	○	○	○	○	○
Limit naps	○	○	○	○	○	○	○
Limit activities in bed	○	○	○	○	○	○	○
Exercise	○	○	○	○	○	○	○
Meditate	○	○	○	○	○	○	○
Journaling	○	○	○	○	○	○	○
No food late night	○	○	○	○	○	○	○
Shut off electronics in the evening	○	○	○	○	○	○	○
Less caffeine	○	○	○	○	○	○	○
Take magnesium	○	○	○	○	○	○	○

MY PRIORITIES FOR THIS WEEK

GRATITUDE LOG

MAIN GOALS

DAILY ACTIVITIES

	M	T	W	T	F	S	S
Follow sleep routine	○	○	○	○	○	○	○
Avoid alcohol	○	○	○	○	○	○	○
Limit naps	○	○	○	○	○	○	○
Limit activities in bed	○	○	○	○	○	○	○
Exercise	○	○	○	○	○	○	○
Meditate	○	○	○	○	○	○	○
Journaling	○	○	○	○	○	○	○
No food late night	○	○	○	○	○	○	○
Shut off electronics in the evening	○	○	○	○	○	○	○
Less caffeine	○	○	○	○	○	○	○
Take magnesium	○	○	○	○	○	○	○

MY PRIORITIES FOR THIS WEEK

GRATITUDE LOG

MAIN GOALS

DAILY ACTIVITIES

	M	T	W	T	F	S	S
Follow sleep routine	○	○	○	○	○	○	○
Avoid alcohol	○	○	○	○	○	○	○
Limit naps	○	○	○	○	○	○	○
Limit activities in bed	○	○	○	○	○	○	○
Exercise	○	○	○	○	○	○	○
Meditate	○	○	○	○	○	○	○
Journaling	○	○	○	○	○	○	○
No food late night	○	○	○	○	○	○	○
Shut off electronics in the evening	○	○	○	○	○	○	○
Less caffeine	○	○	○	○	○	○	○
Take magnesium	○	○	○	○	○	○	○

MY PRIORITIES FOR THIS WEEK

GRATITUDE LOG

MAIN GOALS

DAILY ACTIVITIES

	M	T	W	T	F	S	S
Follow sleep routine	○	○	○	○	○	○	○
Avoid alcohol	○	○	○	○	○	○	○
Limit naps	○	○	○	○	○	○	○
Limit activities in bed	○	○	○	○	○	○	○
Exercise	○	○	○	○	○	○	○
Meditate	○	○	○	○	○	○	○
Journaling	○	○	○	○	○	○	○
No food late night	○	○	○	○	○	○	○
Shut off electronics in the evening	○	○	○	○	○	○	○
Less caffeine	○	○	○	○	○	○	○
Take magnesium	○	○	○	○	○	○	○

MY PRIORITIES FOR THIS WEEK

GRATITUDE LOG

MAIN GOALS

DAILY ACTIVITIES

	M	T	W	T	F	S	S
Follow sleep routine	○	○	○	○	○	○	○
Avoid alcohol	○	○	○	○	○	○	○
Limit naps	○	○	○	○	○	○	○
Limit activities in bed	○	○	○	○	○	○	○
Exercise	○	○	○	○	○	○	○
Meditate	○	○	○	○	○	○	○
Journaling	○	○	○	○	○	○	○
No food late night	○	○	○	○	○	○	○
Shut off electronics in the evening	○	○	○	○	○	○	○
Less caffeine	○	○	○	○	○	○	○
Take magnesium	○	○	○	○	○	○	○

MY PRIORITIES FOR THIS WEEK

GRATITUDE LOG

MAIN GOALS

DAILY ACTIVITIES

	M	T	W	T	F	S	S
Follow sleep routine	○	○	○	○	○	○	○
Avoid alcohol	○	○	○	○	○	○	○
Limit naps	○	○	○	○	○	○	○
Limit activities in bed	○	○	○	○	○	○	○
Exercise	○	○	○	○	○	○	○
Meditate	○	○	○	○	○	○	○
Journaling	○	○	○	○	○	○	○
No food late night	○	○	○	○	○	○	○
Shut off electronics in the evening	○	○	○	○	○	○	○
Less caffeine	○	○	○	○	○	○	○
Take magnesium	○	○	○	○	○	○	○

MY PRIORITIES FOR THIS WEEK

GRATITUDE LOG

MAIN GOALS

DAILY ACTIVITIES

	M	T	W	T	F	S	S
Follow sleep routine	○	○	○	○	○	○	○
Avoid alcohol	○	○	○	○	○	○	○
Limit naps	○	○	○	○	○	○	○
Limit activities in bed	○	○	○	○	○	○	○
Exercise	○	○	○	○	○	○	○
Meditate	○	○	○	○	○	○	○
Journaling	○	○	○	○	○	○	○
No food late night	○	○	○	○	○	○	○
Shut off electronics in the evening	○	○	○	○	○	○	○
Less caffeine	○	○	○	○	○	○	○
Take magnesium	○	○	○	○	○	○	○

MY PRIORITIES FOR THIS WEEK

GRATITUDE LOG

MAIN GOALS

DAILY ACTIVITIES

	M	T	W	T	F	S	S
Follow sleep routine	○	○	○	○	○	○	○
Avoid alcohol	○	○	○	○	○	○	○
Limit naps	○	○	○	○	○	○	○
Limit activities in bed	○	○	○	○	○	○	○
Exercise	○	○	○	○	○	○	○
Meditate	○	○	○	○	○	○	○
Journaling	○	○	○	○	○	○	○
No food late night	○	○	○	○	○	○	○
Shut off electronics in the evening	○	○	○	○	○	○	○
Less caffeine	○	○	○	○	○	○	○
Take magnesium	○	○	○	○	○	○	○

MY PRIORITIES FOR THIS WEEK

GRATITUDE LOG

MAIN GOALS

DAILY ACTIVITIES

	M	T	W	T	F	S	S
Follow sleep routine	○	○	○	○	○	○	○
Avoid alcohol	○	○	○	○	○	○	○
Limit naps	○	○	○	○	○	○	○
Limit activities in bed	○	○	○	○	○	○	○
Exercise	○	○	○	○	○	○	○
Meditate	○	○	○	○	○	○	○
Journaling	○	○	○	○	○	○	○
No food late night	○	○	○	○	○	○	○
Shut off electronics in the evening	○	○	○	○	○	○	○
Less caffeine	○	○	○	○	○	○	○
Take magnesium	○	○	○	○	○	○	○

MY PRIORITIES FOR THIS WEEK

GRATITUDE LOG

MAIN GOALS

DAILY ACTIVITIES

	M	T	W	T	F	S	S
Follow sleep routine	○	○	○	○	○	○	○
Avoid alcohol	○	○	○	○	○	○	○
Limit naps	○	○	○	○	○	○	○
Limit activities in bed	○	○	○	○	○	○	○
Exercise	○	○	○	○	○	○	○
Meditate	○	○	○	○	○	○	○
Journaling	○	○	○	○	○	○	○
No food late night	○	○	○	○	○	○	○
Shut off electronics in the evening	○	○	○	○	○	○	○
Less caffeine	○	○	○	○	○	○	○
Take magnesium	○	○	○	○	○	○	○

MY PRIORITIES FOR THIS WEEK

GRATITUDE LOG

MAIN GOALS

DAILY ACTIVITIES

	M	T	W	T	F	S	S
Follow sleep routine	○	○	○	○	○	○	○
Avoid alcohol	○	○	○	○	○	○	○
Limit naps	○	○	○	○	○	○	○
Limit activities in bed	○	○	○	○	○	○	○
Exercise	○	○	○	○	○	○	○
Meditate	○	○	○	○	○	○	○
Journaling	○	○	○	○	○	○	○
No food late night	○	○	○	○	○	○	○
Shut off electronics in the evening	○	○	○	○	○	○	○
Less caffeine	○	○	○	○	○	○	○
Take magnesium	○	○	○	○	○	○	○

MY PRIORITIES FOR THIS WEEK

GRATITUDE LOG

MAIN GOALS

DAILY ACTIVITIES

	M	T	W	T	F	S	S
Follow sleep routine	○	○	○	○	○	○	○
Avoid alcohol	○	○	○	○	○	○	○
Limit naps	○	○	○	○	○	○	○
Limit activities in bed	○	○	○	○	○	○	○
Exercise	○	○	○	○	○	○	○
Meditate	○	○	○	○	○	○	○
Journaling	○	○	○	○	○	○	○
No food late night	○	○	○	○	○	○	○
Shut off electronics in the evening	○	○	○	○	○	○	○
Less caffeine	○	○	○	○	○	○	○
Take magnesium	○	○	○	○	○	○	○

MY PRIORITIES FOR THIS WEEK

GRATITUDE LOG

MAIN GOALS

DAILY ACTIVITIES

	M	T	W	T	F	S	S
Follow sleep routine	○	○	○	○	○	○	○
Avoid alcohol	○	○	○	○	○	○	○
Limit naps	○	○	○	○	○	○	○
Limit activities in bed	○	○	○	○	○	○	○
Exercise	○	○	○	○	○	○	○
Meditate	○	○	○	○	○	○	○
Journaling	○	○	○	○	○	○	○
No food late night	○	○	○	○	○	○	○
Shut off electronics in the evening	○	○	○	○	○	○	○
Less caffeine	○	○	○	○	○	○	○
Take magnesium	○	○	○	○	○	○	○

MY PRIORITIES FOR THIS WEEK

GRATITUDE LOG

MAIN GOALS

DAILY ACTIVITIES

	M	T	W	T	F	S	S
Follow sleep routine	○	○	○	○	○	○	○
Avoid alcohol	○	○	○	○	○	○	○
Limit naps	○	○	○	○	○	○	○
Limit activities in bed	○	○	○	○	○	○	○
Exercise	○	○	○	○	○	○	○
Meditate	○	○	○	○	○	○	○
Journaling	○	○	○	○	○	○	○
No food late night	○	○	○	○	○	○	○
Shut off electronics in the evening	○	○	○	○	○	○	○
Less caffeine	○	○	○	○	○	○	○
Take magnesium	○	○	○	○	○	○	○

MY PRIORITIES FOR THIS WEEK

GRATITUDE LOG

MAIN GOALS

DAILY ACTIVITIES

	M	T	W	T	F	S	S
Follow sleep routine	○	○	○	○	○	○	○
Avoid alcohol	○	○	○	○	○	○	○
Limit naps	○	○	○	○	○	○	○
Limit activities in bed	○	○	○	○	○	○	○
Exercise	○	○	○	○	○	○	○
Meditate	○	○	○	○	○	○	○
Journaling	○	○	○	○	○	○	○
No food late night	○	○	○	○	○	○	○
Shut off electronics in the evening	○	○	○	○	○	○	○
Less caffeine	○	○	○	○	○	○	○
Take magnesium	○	○	○	○	○	○	○

MY PRIORITIES FOR THIS WEEK

GRATITUDE LOG

MAIN GOALS

DAILY ACTIVITIES

	M	T	W	T	F	S	S
Follow sleep routine	○	○	○	○	○	○	○
Avoid alcohol	○	○	○	○	○	○	○
Limit naps	○	○	○	○	○	○	○
Limit activities in bed	○	○	○	○	○	○	○
Exercise	○	○	○	○	○	○	○
Meditate	○	○	○	○	○	○	○
Journaling	○	○	○	○	○	○	○
No food late night	○	○	○	○	○	○	○
Shut off electronics in the evening	○	○	○	○	○	○	○
Less caffeine	○	○	○	○	○	○	○
Take magnesium	○	○	○	○	○	○	○

MY PRIORITIES FOR THIS WEEK

GRATITUDE LOG

MAIN GOALS

DAILY ACTIVITIES

	M	T	W	T	F	S	S
Follow sleep routine	○	○	○	○	○	○	○
Avoid alcohol	○	○	○	○	○	○	○
Limit naps	○	○	○	○	○	○	○
Limit activities in bed	○	○	○	○	○	○	○
Exercise	○	○	○	○	○	○	○
Meditate	○	○	○	○	○	○	○
Journaling	○	○	○	○	○	○	○
No food late night	○	○	○	○	○	○	○
Shut off electronics in the evening	○	○	○	○	○	○	○
Less caffeine	○	○	○	○	○	○	○
Take magnesium	○	○	○	○	○	○	○

MY PRIORITIES FOR THIS WEEK

GRATITUDE LOG

MAIN GOALS

DAILY ACTIVITIES

	M	T	W	T	F	S	S
Follow sleep routine	◯	◯	◯	◯	◯	◯	◯
Avoid alcohol	◯	◯	◯	◯	◯	◯	◯
Limit naps	◯	◯	◯	◯	◯	◯	◯
Limit activities in bed	◯	◯	◯	◯	◯	◯	◯
Exercise	◯	◯	◯	◯	◯	◯	◯
Meditate	◯	◯	◯	◯	◯	◯	◯
Journaling	◯	◯	◯	◯	◯	◯	◯
No food late night	◯	◯	◯	◯	◯	◯	◯
Shut off electronics in the evening	◯	◯	◯	◯	◯	◯	◯
Less caffeine	◯	◯	◯	◯	◯	◯	◯
Take magnesium	◯	◯	◯	◯	◯	◯	◯

MY PRIORITIES FOR THIS WEEK

GRATITUDE LOG

MAIN GOALS

DAILY ACTIVITIES

	M	T	W	T	F	S	S
Follow sleep routine	○	○	○	○	○	○	○
Avoid alcohol	○	○	○	○	○	○	○
Limit naps	○	○	○	○	○	○	○
Limit activities in bed	○	○	○	○	○	○	○
Exercise	○	○	○	○	○	○	○
Meditate	○	○	○	○	○	○	○
Journaling	○	○	○	○	○	○	○
No food late night	○	○	○	○	○	○	○
Shut off electronics in the evening	○	○	○	○	○	○	○
Less caffeine	○	○	○	○	○	○	○
Take magnesium	○	○	○	○	○	○	○

MY PRIORITIES FOR THIS WEEK

GRATITUDE LOG

MAIN GOALS

DAILY ACTIVITIES

	M	T	W	T	F	S	S
Follow sleep routine	○	○	○	○	○	○	○
Avoid alcohol	○	○	○	○	○	○	○
Limit naps	○	○	○	○	○	○	○
Limit activities in bed	○	○	○	○	○	○	○
Exercise	○	○	○	○	○	○	○
Meditate	○	○	○	○	○	○	○
Journaling	○	○	○	○	○	○	○
No food late night	○	○	○	○	○	○	○
Shut off electronics in the evening	○	○	○	○	○	○	○
Less caffeine	○	○	○	○	○	○	○
Take magnesium	○	○	○	○	○	○	○

MY PRIORITIES FOR THIS WEEK

GRATITUDE LOG

MAIN GOALS

DAILY ACTIVITIES

	M	T	W	T	F	S	S
Follow sleep routine	○	○	○	○	○	○	○
Avoid alcohol	○	○	○	○	○	○	○
Limit naps	○	○	○	○	○	○	○
Limit activities in bed	○	○	○	○	○	○	○
Exercise	○	○	○	○	○	○	○
Meditate	○	○	○	○	○	○	○
Journaling	○	○	○	○	○	○	○
No food late night	○	○	○	○	○	○	○
Shut off electronics in the evening	○	○	○	○	○	○	○
Less caffeine	○	○	○	○	○	○	○
Take magnesium	○	○	○	○	○	○	○

MY PRIORITIES FOR THIS WEEK

GRATITUDE LOG

MAIN GOALS

DAILY ACTIVITIES

	M	T	W	T	F	S	S
Follow sleep routine	○	○	○	○	○	○	○
Avoid alcohol	○	○	○	○	○	○	○
Limit naps	○	○	○	○	○	○	○
Limit activities in bed	○	○	○	○	○	○	○
Exercise	○	○	○	○	○	○	○
Meditate	○	○	○	○	○	○	○
Journaling	○	○	○	○	○	○	○
No food late night	○	○	○	○	○	○	○
Shut off electronics in the evening	○	○	○	○	○	○	○
Less caffeine	○	○	○	○	○	○	○
Take magnesium	○	○	○	○	○	○	○

MY PRIORITIES FOR THIS WEEK

GRATITUDE LOG

MAIN GOALS

DAILY ACTIVITIES

	M	T	W	T	F	S	S
Follow sleep routine	○	○	○	○	○	○	○
Avoid alcohol	○	○	○	○	○	○	○
Limit naps	○	○	○	○	○	○	○
Limit activities in bed	○	○	○	○	○	○	○
Exercise	○	○	○	○	○	○	○
Meditate	○	○	○	○	○	○	○
Journaling	○	○	○	○	○	○	○
No food late night	○	○	○	○	○	○	○
Shut off electronics in the evening	○	○	○	○	○	○	○
Less caffeine	○	○	○	○	○	○	○
Take magnesium	○	○	○	○	○	○	○

MY PRIORITIES FOR THIS WEEK

GRATITUDE LOG

MAIN GOALS

DAILY ACTIVITIES

	M	T	W	T	F	S	S
Follow sleep routine	○	○	○	○	○	○	○
Avoid alcohol	○	○	○	○	○	○	○
Limit naps	○	○	○	○	○	○	○
Limit activities in bed	○	○	○	○	○	○	○
Exercise	○	○	○	○	○	○	○
Meditate	○	○	○	○	○	○	○
Journaling	○	○	○	○	○	○	○
No food late night	○	○	○	○	○	○	○
Shut off electronics in the evening	○	○	○	○	○	○	○
Less caffeine	○	○	○	○	○	○	○
Take magnesium	○	○	○	○	○	○	○

MY PRIORITIES FOR THIS WEEK

GRATITUDE LOG

MAIN GOALS

DAILY ACTIVITIES

	M	T	W	T	F	S	S
Follow sleep routine	○	○	○	○	○	○	○
Avoid alcohol	○	○	○	○	○	○	○
Limit naps	○	○	○	○	○	○	○
Limit activities in bed	○	○	○	○	○	○	○
Exercise	○	○	○	○	○	○	○
Meditate	○	○	○	○	○	○	○
Journaling	○	○	○	○	○	○	○
No food late night	○	○	○	○	○	○	○
Shut off electronics in the evening	○	○	○	○	○	○	○
Less caffeine	○	○	○	○	○	○	○
Take magnesium	○	○	○	○	○	○	○

MY PRIORITIES FOR THIS WEEK

GRATITUDE LOG

MAIN GOALS

DAILY ACTIVITIES

	M	T	W	T	F	S	S
Follow sleep routine	○	○	○	○	○	○	○
Avoid alcohol	○	○	○	○	○	○	○
Limit naps	○	○	○	○	○	○	○
Limit activities in bed	○	○	○	○	○	○	○
Exercise	○	○	○	○	○	○	○
Meditate	○	○	○	○	○	○	○
Journaling	○	○	○	○	○	○	○
No food late night	○	○	○	○	○	○	○
Shut off electronics in the evening	○	○	○	○	○	○	○
Less caffeine	○	○	○	○	○	○	○
Take magnesium	○	○	○	○	○	○	○

MY PRIORITIES FOR THIS WEEK

GRATITUDE LOG

MAIN GOALS

DAILY ACTIVITIES

	M	T	W	T	F	S	S
Follow sleep routine	○	○	○	○	○	○	○
Avoid alcohol	○	○	○	○	○	○	○
Limit naps	○	○	○	○	○	○	○
Limit activities in bed	○	○	○	○	○	○	○
Exercise	○	○	○	○	○	○	○
Meditate	○	○	○	○	○	○	○
Journaling	○	○	○	○	○	○	○
No food late night	○	○	○	○	○	○	○
Shut off electronics in the evening	○	○	○	○	○	○	○
Less caffeine	○	○	○	○	○	○	○
Take magnesium	○	○	○	○	○	○	○

MY PRIORITIES FOR THIS WEEK

GRATITUDE LOG

MAIN GOALS

DAILY ACTIVITIES

	M	T	W	T	F	S	S
Follow sleep routine	○	○	○	○	○	○	○
Avoid alcohol	○	○	○	○	○	○	○
Limit naps	○	○	○	○	○	○	○
Limit activities in bed	○	○	○	○	○	○	○
Exercise	○	○	○	○	○	○	○
Meditate	○	○	○	○	○	○	○
Journaling	○	○	○	○	○	○	○
No food late night	○	○	○	○	○	○	○
Shut off electronics in the evening	○	○	○	○	○	○	○
Less caffeine	○	○	○	○	○	○	○
Take magnesium	○	○	○	○	○	○	○

MY PRIORITIES FOR THIS WEEK

GRATITUDE LOG

MAIN GOALS

DAILY ACTIVITIES

	M	T	W	T	F	S	S
Follow sleep routine	○	○	○	○	○	○	○
Avoid alcohol	○	○	○	○	○	○	○
Limit naps	○	○	○	○	○	○	○
Limit activities in bed	○	○	○	○	○	○	○
Exercise	○	○	○	○	○	○	○
Meditate	○	○	○	○	○	○	○
Journaling	○	○	○	○	○	○	○
No food late night	○	○	○	○	○	○	○
Shut off electronics in the evening	○	○	○	○	○	○	○
Less caffeine	○	○	○	○	○	○	○
Take magnesium	○	○	○	○	○	○	○

MY PRIORITIES FOR THIS WEEK

GRATITUDE LOG

MAIN GOALS

DAILY ACTIVITIES

	M	T	W	T	F	S	S
Follow sleep routine	○	○	○	○	○	○	○
Avoid alcohol	○	○	○	○	○	○	○
Limit naps	○	○	○	○	○	○	○
Limit activities in bed	○	○	○	○	○	○	○
Exercise	○	○	○	○	○	○	○
Meditate	○	○	○	○	○	○	○
Journaling	○	○	○	○	○	○	○
No food late night	○	○	○	○	○	○	○
Shut off electronics in the evening	○	○	○	○	○	○	○
Less caffeine	○	○	○	○	○	○	○
Take magnesium	○	○	○	○	○	○	○

MY PRIORITIES FOR THIS WEEK

GRATITUDE LOG

MAIN GOALS

DAILY ACTIVITIES

	M	T	W	T	F	S	S
Follow sleep routine	○	○	○	○	○	○	○
Avoid alcohol	○	○	○	○	○	○	○
Limit naps	○	○	○	○	○	○	○
Limit activities in bed	○	○	○	○	○	○	○
Exercise	○	○	○	○	○	○	○
Meditate	○	○	○	○	○	○	○
Journaling	○	○	○	○	○	○	○
No food late night	○	○	○	○	○	○	○
Shut off electronics in the evening	○	○	○	○	○	○	○
Less caffeine	○	○	○	○	○	○	○
Take magnesium	○	○	○	○	○	○	○

MY PRIORITIES FOR THIS WEEK

GRATITUDE LOG

MAIN GOALS

DAILY ACTIVITIES

	M	T	W	T	F	S	S
Follow sleep routine	○	○	○	○	○	○	○
Avoid alcohol	○	○	○	○	○	○	○
Limit naps	○	○	○	○	○	○	○
Limit activities in bed	○	○	○	○	○	○	○
Exercise	○	○	○	○	○	○	○
Meditate	○	○	○	○	○	○	○
Journaling	○	○	○	○	○	○	○
No food late night	○	○	○	○	○	○	○
Shut off electronics in the evening	○	○	○	○	○	○	○
Less caffeine	○	○	○	○	○	○	○
Take magnesium	○	○	○	○	○	○	○

MY PRIORITIES FOR THIS WEEK

GRATITUDE LOG

MAIN GOALS

DAILY ACTIVITIES

	M	T	W	T	F	S	S
Follow sleep routine	○	○	○	○	○	○	○
Avoid alcohol	○	○	○	○	○	○	○
Limit naps	○	○	○	○	○	○	○
Limit activities in bed	○	○	○	○	○	○	○
Exercise	○	○	○	○	○	○	○
Meditate	○	○	○	○	○	○	○
Journaling	○	○	○	○	○	○	○
No food late night	○	○	○	○	○	○	○
Shut off electronics in the evening	○	○	○	○	○	○	○
Less caffeine	○	○	○	○	○	○	○
Take magnesium	○	○	○	○	○	○	○

MY PRIORITIES FOR THIS WEEK

GRATITUDE LOG

MAIN GOALS

DAILY ACTIVITIES

	M	T	W	T	F	S	S
Follow sleep routine	○	○	○	○	○	○	○
Avoid alcohol	○	○	○	○	○	○	○
Limit naps	○	○	○	○	○	○	○
Limit activities in bed	○	○	○	○	○	○	○
Exercise	○	○	○	○	○	○	○
Meditate	○	○	○	○	○	○	○
Journaling	○	○	○	○	○	○	○
No food late night	○	○	○	○	○	○	○
Shut off electronics in the evening	○	○	○	○	○	○	○
Less caffeine	○	○	○	○	○	○	○
Take magnesium	○	○	○	○	○	○	○

MY PRIORITIES FOR THIS WEEK

GRATITUDE LOG

MAIN GOALS

DAILY ACTIVITIES

	M	T	W	T	F	S	S
Follow sleep routine	○	○	○	○	○	○	○
Avoid alcohol	○	○	○	○	○	○	○
Limit naps	○	○	○	○	○	○	○
Limit activities in bed	○	○	○	○	○	○	○
Exercise	○	○	○	○	○	○	○
Meditate	○	○	○	○	○	○	○
Journaling	○	○	○	○	○	○	○
No food late night	○	○	○	○	○	○	○
Shut off electronics in the evening	○	○	○	○	○	○	○
Less caffeine	○	○	○	○	○	○	○
Take magnesium	○	○	○	○	○	○	○

MY PRIORITIES FOR THIS WEEK

GRATITUDE LOG

MAIN GOALS

DAILY ACTIVITIES

	M	T	W	T	F	S	S
Follow sleep routine	◯	◯	◯	◯	◯	◯	◯
Avoid alcohol	◯	◯	◯	◯	◯	◯	◯
Limit naps	◯	◯	◯	◯	◯	◯	◯
Limit activities in bed	◯	◯	◯	◯	◯	◯	◯
Exercise	◯	◯	◯	◯	◯	◯	◯
Meditate	◯	◯	◯	◯	◯	◯	◯
Journaling	◯	◯	◯	◯	◯	◯	◯
No food late night	◯	◯	◯	◯	◯	◯	◯
Shut off electronics in the evening	◯	◯	◯	◯	◯	◯	◯
Less caffeine	◯	◯	◯	◯	◯	◯	◯
Take magnesium	◯	◯	◯	◯	◯	◯	◯

MY PRIORITIES FOR THIS WEEK

GRATITUDE LOG

MAIN GOALS

DAILY ACTIVITIES

	M	T	W	T	F	S	S
Follow sleep routine	○	○	○	○	○	○	○
Avoid alcohol	○	○	○	○	○	○	○
Limit naps	○	○	○	○	○	○	○
Limit activities in bed	○	○	○	○	○	○	○
Exercise	○	○	○	○	○	○	○
Meditate	○	○	○	○	○	○	○
Journaling	○	○	○	○	○	○	○
No food late night	○	○	○	○	○	○	○
Shut off electronics in the evening	○	○	○	○	○	○	○
Less caffeine	○	○	○	○	○	○	○
Take magnesium	○	○	○	○	○	○	○

MY PRIORITIES FOR THIS WEEK

GRATITUDE LOG

MAIN GOALS

DAILY ACTIVITIES

	M	T	W	T	F	S	S
Follow sleep routine	○	○	○	○	○	○	○
Avoid alcohol	○	○	○	○	○	○	○
Limit naps	○	○	○	○	○	○	○
Limit activities in bed	○	○	○	○	○	○	○
Exercise	○	○	○	○	○	○	○
Meditate	○	○	○	○	○	○	○
Journaling	○	○	○	○	○	○	○
No food late night	○	○	○	○	○	○	○
Shut off electronics in the evening	○	○	○	○	○	○	○
Less caffeine	○	○	○	○	○	○	○
Take magnesium	○	○	○	○	○	○	○

MY PRIORITIES FOR THIS WEEK

GRATITUDE LOG

MAIN GOALS

DAILY ACTIVITIES

	M	T	W	T	F	S	S
Follow sleep routine	○	○	○	○	○	○	○
Avoid alcohol	○	○	○	○	○	○	○
Limit naps	○	○	○	○	○	○	○
Limit activities in bed	○	○	○	○	○	○	○
Exercise	○	○	○	○	○	○	○
Meditate	○	○	○	○	○	○	○
Journaling	○	○	○	○	○	○	○
No food late night	○	○	○	○	○	○	○
Shut off electronics in the evening	○	○	○	○	○	○	○
Less caffeine	○	○	○	○	○	○	○
Take magnesium	○	○	○	○	○	○	○